THE BIPOLAR SURVIVAL
WORKBOOK

THE BIPOLAR SURVIVAL WORKBOOK

LIVING WITH AND OVERCOMING BIPOLAR DISORDER

Dr Steven Thomas

Distributed by SwordWorks Books, UK

ISBN 978-1-906512-36-1

FOREWORD

Bipolar Disorder is regarded by many as a scourge of the modern world. First diagnosed during the 19th century by a French psychiatrist, the disorder has caused a great deal of misery for many people. The disorder is of course characterised by mood swings to opposite poles of mania and depression. Between these two extremes sufferers of one experience periods when their symptoms appear to have gone away, often a danger time when patients with extreme symptoms cease taking their medication because they "feel better". The disease itself can cause massive disruption not only to the sufferer but to their family, friends and colleagues as well. In very extreme cases attempts of suicide and similar instances of extreme harm can be a characteristic of this disorder.

The incredible disruption of living one's life from extremes of clinical depression to heights of manic activity when insomnia can last for several nights in succession can only be imagined by those people who have not experienced it. It is of course essential that people who feel they may be suffering from these kinds of symptoms should seek professional advice and treatment in the first instance. However, Bipolar Disorder is not an illness that can always be treated to the extent that it completely goes away. The purpose of this book is to work with a range of therapies to produce a combined approach that will suit individuals, rather than offer a "one size fits all" approach that will be unsuitable for very many patients.

The type of therapies covered in this book could generally be categorised as holistic, in that they treat a wider range of symptoms and conditions than the pure instances of depression and mania. For example, the benefits of exercise are well-known for increasing mood, including an instant release of serotonin in the brain that is better than any prescribed drug could possibly be. Added to the benefits in self-esteem experienced by the person exercising and you have a recipe for success. Does this directly treat the Bipolar Disorder? Possibly the release of serotonin is helpful in a direct sense, but the real benefit is that added to a great number of other therapies which we will explore in this book the exercise itself is just one building block in a whole structure that will become an extremely valuable route to recovering good health, happiness and well-being.

We hope and trust that you will work through all of the therapies that we have to offer in this book. It is unlikely that all of them will work for you, and they are by no means definitive. The most successful patients will be the ones who are the most active in seeking to find the kind of therapies that suit their personality, lifestyle, emotional makeup, physiological makeup, in other words that fit themselves as a whole person.

In starting this book you have taken an extremely important step on the road to recovery from the worst effects of Bipolar Disorder, if not a total recovery itself which will be possible in many cases. We wish you the very best of luck and the very best of health.

CONTENTS

CONTENTS

INTRODUCTION

Is there a single treatment for Bipolar Disorder? The emotional disorder formerly known as manic depression that seems to have swept through the western world causing untold misery and destruction to the lives of sufferers. We do not believe that there is as such a magic bullet. Clearly in the case of people who are deeply emotionally troubled, there may be no clear alternative to the prospect of prescribed medication to deal with the worst of their symptoms, at least in the short term. In this respect there may well be no clear alternative to advice from a professional therapist who will advise the patient accordingly and may or may not describe a course of medication. The object of this book is to show that the different methods of treating Bipolar Disorder, which have proved successful in a great number of cases.

Indeed, drug therapy itself is by no means a guaranteed path to being cured of Bipolar Disorder. There is no doubt that many sufferers, especially those who have the most severe symptoms, had been treated with drugs to the extent that their moods stabilised and they are able to live or less normal life. But what about the majority of sufferers who may be in the very early stages of Bipolar Disorder or may be suffering from the symptoms in a much less severe and more controllable manner? We believe that this great mass of people is not necessarily best served by automatically reaching for the prescription pad. Instead, we feel that the sufferer needs to be aware of a whole range of different options that can be used in their treatment, with or without drugs.

As we outlined in the foreword, this holistic type of approach is required that the patient explore a wide range of therapies to find which one is most suited to them. These are not normal and untested ideas. The effects of diet and exercise on mood had been well researched and documented on numerous occasions and their therapeutic benefit is beyond doubt. There is currently a great deal of concern in the western world about diet, together with attention that is being focused on food additives. There has been wide research on the effects of both food additives and allergies with varying results on patients with emotional disorders. One thing is clear, the benefits of exploring the question of diet, food additives and allergies is vital as part of the combined approach to curing Bipolar Disorder. There are countless stories of patients with extreme emotional disorders and the psychosis that have successfully changed their diet, removing the foodstuff or additive that appears to be causing their problems, and resulting in a complete remission of symptoms. The word here is complete, not partial. In many cases there is conclusive evidence that one single foodstuff or allergy as being sufficient itself to cause the severe problems that were the original complaint.

Yet another therapy that is gaining a great deal of credence is Cognitive Behavioural Therapy. When this particular therapy was initially developed it was frowned on by a number of professionals and regarded as being part of "crank" medicine. Yet Cognitive Behavioural Therapy, or CBT, is gaining ground and admirers at a very rapid rate. The reason for this is quite simple. The therapy works. Not in every case, there are some people who just do not seem to respond to CBT. Just as there are some people that do not appear to derive any worthwhile benefits from medication.

That is why this book is so important. We recognise that people are different, that people's symptoms are different, and that often the reasons for people having this kind of illness are different. We are dealing with children, young adults, mature adults and the elderly. All of these require different treatments and approaches. That is what we offer in this book, a range of therapies that you can use it yourself and adapt to your own circumstances.

This is not a simple path that you have embarked upon. But it is probably the most important path in your life that you have ever undertaken, especially if you intend to live a positive, happy and well adjusted lifestyle. Many people do recover, some fairly quickly and others over a longer period. The important factor here is that you concentrate on the word "recovery". As soon as you embark on the various therapies outlined in this book there is no question that your recovery is beginning.

Just reading this book is itself a positive step. Your recovery will not happen by itself, or at least it is unlikely to. The more you do your utmost to take steps to bring about your recovery of health and well-being, the faster it will happen. And of course there is the tremendous plus that with every single little step that you take you will fall that little bit better. We will do our utmost to help you build on these little steps, and trust that you will do your utmost to do them justice.

Dr. Steven Thomas

CHAPTER ONE

BIPOLAR DISORDER

"Success is to be measured not so much by the position that one has reached in life... as by the obstacles which he has overcome while trying to succeed."

Booker T. Washington

Before we look into the question of how to deal with Bipolar Disorder lets take a long hard look at the illness itself so that we fully understand what we are dealing with. Bipolar Disorder has also been known in the past as Manic Depression, or Manic Depressive Disorder. These days these days it is more normal and indeed considered more polite to refer to the illness as bipolar disorder. The illness itself is the result of a psychiatric diagnosis of certain mood disorders that contribute to the existence of the illness of bipolar disorder itself. In practice the illness exists where the presence of alternating episodes of abnormally elevated mood, sometimes known as mania, cycle with depressive episodes. It is often the case that between the extreme cycles of mania and depression the patient can experience periods of relative calmness, although it is equally, if not more so for patients to suffer from rapid cycling, where they experience manic episodes and depressive episodes in quick succession. In its most serious state the disorder of bipolar illness can occasionally lead to psychotic symptoms, these can take the form of such things as delusions and hallucinations.

Fortunately Bipolar Disorder is still relatively uncommon, although as many as 1% of the population can suffer from full bipolar disorder at some stage during their lives, and as many as 5% suffer from a less severe form. The more severe forms of Bipolar Disorder are generally experienced, or at least the initial onset of symptoms is experienced, early in life, either in late childhood or during early adult life. Sufferers generally seek help, or are encouraged to seek help, and are able to report their symptoms. Frequently the disorder is reported or the patient seeks treatment at a stage when they are considerably distressed, or the lives and the lives of those around them have suffered quite major disruption. There is even an increased risk of suicide in certain patients, especially after a prolonged period of Bipolar Disorder and during the depressive phase of the illness.

The cause of Bipolar Disorder is not entirely known. Genetic factors have been shown to be a contributory part of the development of Bipolar Disorder. The full extent of how environmental factors contribute towards the onset of the disease, as opposed to genetic factors, is still unknown. However what is known is that there is a quite definite link between certain environmental factors and the onset of the disorder. Conventional treatment for bipolar disorder is with medication, or at least generally with medication, and certainly in the more severe cases. Another treatment that has been used with some considerable success is psychotherapy, although this tends to be used during the less severe stages of the disorder. At the other extreme bipolar sufferers can be committed to hospital on an involuntary basis where it is felt that they present a danger to themselves or to others. One such danger would clearly be where during the depressive phase of the illness the sufferer exhibits suicidal tendencies.

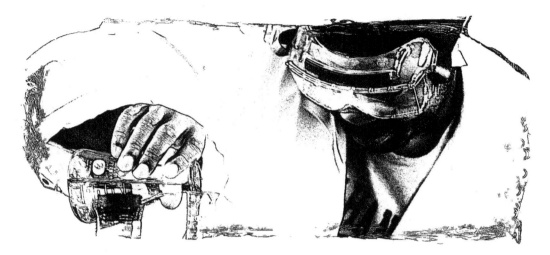

The conventional view of sufferers of Bipolar Disorder is unfortunately not a happy one, with considerable prejudice and disfavour being shown to people suffering this disease. Bipolar sufferers often feel that, as well as their disease, they are labouring under the additional obstacle of extreme social stigma. They are occasionally mistaken for schizophrenics. Although Schizophrenia is an illness that may appear to some to have similarities with Bipolar Disorder, it is in no way the same illness. Bipolar Disorder was first identified during the 19th century, and identified as manic depressive illness by the German psychiatrist Emil Krapaelin. During the 20th century the illness was the subject of considerable research and in the 1950s began to be described as Bipolar disorder.

How do we identify Bipolar Disorder? Put simply, it is a condition in which sufferers experience unusually animated moods, the manic phase of the illness, followed by unusually depressed moods, the depressive phase of the illness. These phases can last for a differing periods. There are no hard and fast rules as to how long each phase lasts and whether or not certain sufferers will have periods of relief in between the two extremes. Bipolar Disorder can be suffered equally by men and women and certainly has not been identified as being any more prevalent in any particular ethnic group. Apart from the aforementioned causes that have been identified, further research suggests that Bipolar Disorder could be rooted in some way in certain chemical imbalances in the brain.

Manic episodes can cause people to:-

- feel wonderful as if nothing could go wrong
- be very agitated and short fused

- be uncooperative and belligerent
- be overly angry and aggressive
- talk too fast or take constantly risky or impulsive actions
- be sexual promiscuous
- have spending binges
- have little sleep
- be easily distracted and unable to stay focused
- having a feeling of great self worth or invincibility
- become too focused on a goal
- have racing thoughts

Depressive episodes can cause:-

- depression and sadness
- loss of interest or wanting to do anything
- no longer enjoying the things one used to do for fun
- loss of weight without being on a diet
- decrease or increase in appetite
- insomnia or restlessness
- feeling sluggish or excessive sleeping
- constant fatigue or loss of energy
- feeling worthless or inappropriately or excessively guilty
- difficulty thinking, concentrating and making decisions
- thoughts of suicide, making a suicide plan, or actually making an attempt

The typical sufferer experiences phases of sadness, anxiety, guilt, anger, isolation and hopelessness. Severe insomnia is by no means unusual in sufferers. Changes in appetite, increased fatigue and increasing degrees of apathy manifest themselves very commonly. Typically sufferers will have problems concentrating, will feel lonely, degrees of self-loathing, apathy or indifference and a lot of interest in sexual activities. They are often shy people, awkward in social situations and at the same time subject to fits of irritability. Chronic pain is another reported factor in the illness and, as already stated, extreme cases show that the sufferer can feel suicidal on occasion.

One of the more encouraging treatments for Bipolar Disorder is Cognitive Behaviour Therapy (CBT). Used frequently in the treatment of depressive illness, CBT has increasingly been shown to help bipolar sufferers, during both the manic and the depressive states, to live more normal and less stressful lives and indeed to decrease the incidents and likelihood of further attacks. The outlook is not totally gloomy however. We intend to examine a range of options that will help you at the very least to manage Bipolar Disorder and at best will hopefully assist you to rid yourself of many, if not all, of the symptoms that you suffer. What is essential is that you take action, such as you are doing now by reading this book. Educating yourself about the illness is not of course enough. Action means a range of activities that will all help you to overcome the problem. Here are some things that you can do initially to begin mitigating the worst problems of the illness.

As well as educating yourself about the disorder:-

- Talk to other people who have had experience of it and find out what kinds of therapies work for them.
- Find a therapist. If necessary try several before deciding on the one that best suits you.
- Do your best to identify and recognise the early warning signs of an impending relapse, have a plan ready to deal with this relapse. In many cases this action plan can avoid the attack altogether.
- Find a friend to help with your problems, someone that can advise you when you may not realise that your mental state is deteriorating.
- Work with your family and friends to help you get over the illness.
- Remember to always take medication when prescribed, if you have any doubts about this you must discuss them with your medical practitioner.
- Again, if you are unhappy with your medication, perhaps feel that it is not working for you, discuss it with your doctor before stopping the medication.
- Take regular exercise and do your best to eat nutritious healthy food on a regular basis
- Aim to establish a regular sleeping pattern.
- Absolutely avoid artificial stimulants and depressants. Coffee, alcohol and of course all illegal drugs are a very bad idea for Bipolar Disorder sufferers.

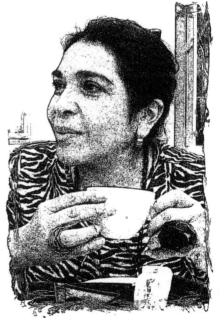

If you are reading this book as a family member or friend of a bipolar sufferer there are many things that you can do to help this person. Firstly, let them know that you have noticed a change in their behaviour, and suggest that they should consider seeking help from a professional if they are enthusiastic on regaining their quality of life. Remind the sufferer to take their medication as and when prescribed. Keep a watchful eye on the sufferer's mood, so that you can be aware of mood swings at the very start of their onset, and give the sufferer as much a warning and support as possible. You can of course work with the sufferer to help them with their action plans to deal with the illness, as well as help them draw up such things as exercise and healthy eating plans that will aid them in their recovery, or at the very least to mitigate the worst effects of the illness. Try and keep yourself abreast of all current developments in the bipolar field. You could well consider joining a bipolar family support group or just keep in touch with the sufferer's therapist so that you are best equipped to help deal with the problem.

> *"So I feel that I may be suffering from bipolar disorder, or somebody I know may be suffering from Bipolar Disorder, how can I confirm this one way or the other? "*

The complete answer of course is it that if you suspect that this may be the case, it is essential that you contact a qualified medical practitioner and obtain a professional diagnosis. Once you are in possession of this diagnosis, and with the accompanying advice and possible medication that will accompany it, you are on the path to beginning the battle to come to terms with and defeat the illness. Initially, we have a simple diagnostic questionnaire that you could fear then and at least get some indication as to whether or not you may be a sufferer.

THE MOOD DISORDER QUESTIONNAIRE

Instructions: Please answer each question to the best of your ability.

1. Has there ever been a period of time when you were not your usual self and …	YES	NO
…you felt so good or so hyper that other people thought you were not your Normal self or you were so hyper that you got into trouble?		
…you were so irritable that you shouted at people or started fights or arguments?		
…you felt much more self-confident than usual?		
…you got much less sleep than usual and found you didn't really miss it?		
…you were much more talkative or spoke much faster than usual?		
… thoughts raced through your head or you couldn't slow your mind down?		
…you were so easily distracted by things around you that you had trouble concentrating or staying on track?		
… you had much more energy than usual?		
… you were much more active or did many more things than usual?		
… you were much more social or outgoing than usual, for example, you telephoned friends in the middle of the night?		
… you were much more interested in sex than usual?		
… you did things that were unusual for you or that other people might have thought were excessive, foolish, or risky?		
… spending money got you or your family into trouble?		
2. If you checked YES to more than one of the above, have several of these ever happened during the same period of time?		
3. How much of a problem did any of these cause you -like being unable to work; having family, money or legal troubles; getting into arguments or fights? Please circle one response only.		
5. Has a health professional ever told you that you have manic-depressive illness or bipolar disorder?		

You can try filling in the questionnaire and see how many positive responses you make to the questions. If you feel that more than half of your responses are positive, then you really should be seeking some sort of medical advice. If your positive responses are less than 50% you should still consider that you clearly have some underlying reason for feeling that you have a problem and you should discuss your symptoms with your doctor.

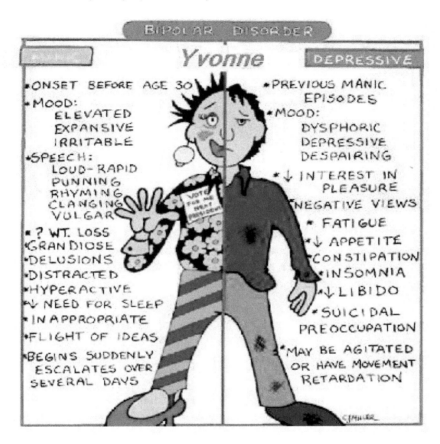

You should know the difference between psychopharmacologists, psychiatrists, psychotherapists, social workers and counsellors. It's a new world, and confusing to the uninitiated. Here is a short list of some of the professions you'll encounter:-

Psychopharmacologists are psychiatrists who have two additional years of training after completing medical school and then a psychiatric residency. These extra years are devoted to learning brain chemistry and how various medications interact. If you are lucky, your medical plan will allow you to see one. They can be very expensive but worth it if you find a good one.

Psychiatrists are doctors who, after medical school, serve a residency in a psychiatric setting.

It used to be that psychiatrists were into Freud, Jung and/or Adler and years were wasted talking about your id or white rats or whatever. Very few practice that form of therapy any longer. You now most likely will see a psychiatrist for diagnosis and medical treatment.

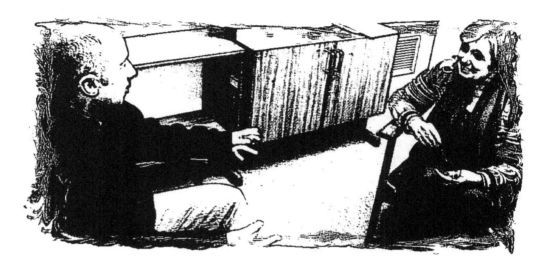

Psychotherapists are people trained in helping other people resolve issues related to depression. They are not really much help to a person with Bipolar Disorder unless or until the Bipolar Disorder is under control. Only then can a person with Bipolar Disorder benefit from this type of therapy.

Counsellors are people trained in short-term counselling, helping people find out what their problems are and helping them resolve them in the short-term. Usually they can also refer the person they are seeing to whatever or whoever they need to in order to seek help with problems which cannot be resolved in the short term.

Social workers can cover many areas. Usually subjects covered by a psychotherapist, can act as a counsellor and can act as an agent to help people in need connect with the services that will help them resolve their difficulties.

Counsellors and social workers are the least easily defined category because they both can conceivably cover quite a large territory, depending upon what their job entails, who it is they work for, if they are in private practice, etc.

More than two million American adults, around 1% of the adult population any given year, have Bipolar Disorder. Bipolar disorder typically develops in late adolescence or early adulthood. However, some people have their first symptoms during childhood, some develop them late in life. It is often not recognised as an illness and people may suffer for years before it is properly diagnosed and treated. Like diabetes or heart disease, Bipolar Disorder is a long-term illness that must be carefully managed throughout a person's life.

"Manic-depression distorts moods and thoughts, incites dreadful behaviours, destroys the basis of rational thought and too often erodes the desire and will to live. It is an illness that is biological in its origins, yet one that feels psychological in the experience of it; an illness that is unique in conferring advantage and pleasure, yet one that brings in its wake almost unendurable suffering and, not infrequently, suicide.

I am fortunate that I have not died from my illness, fortunate in having received the best medical care available, and fortunate in having the friends, colleagues, and family that I do."

Bipolar disorder causes dramatic mood swings—from overly high and/or irritable to sad and hopeless, and then back again, often with periods of normal mood in between. Severe changes in energy and behaviour can accompany with these changes in mood. The periods of highs and lows are called episodes of mania and depression.

- Signs and symptoms of mania (or a manic episode) include:-
- increased energy, activity, and restlessness
- excessively high, overly good, euphoric mood
- extreme irritability
- racing thoughts and talking very fast, jumping from one idea to another
- distractibility, can't concentrate well
- little sleep needed
- unrealistic beliefs in one's abilities and powers
- poor judgment
- spending sprees
- a lasting period of behaviour that is different from usual
- increased sexual drive
- abuse of drugs (particularly cocaine), alcohol, and sleeping medications
- provocative, intrusive or aggressive behaviour
- denial that anything is wrong

A manic episode is diagnosed if elevated mood occurs with three or more of the other symptoms most of the day, nearly every day, for one week or longer. If the mood is irritable, four additional symptoms must be present.

Signs and symptoms of depression (or a depressive episode) include:-

- lasting sad, anxious or empty mood
- feelings of hopelessness or pessimism
- feelings of guilt, worthlessness or helplessness

- loss of interest or pleasure in activities once enjoyed, including sex
- decreased energy, a feeling of fatigue or of being "slowed down"
- difficulty concentrating, remembering and making decisions
- restlessness or irritability
- sleeping too much, or unable to sleep
- change in appetite and/or unintended weight loss or gain
- chronic pain or other persistent bodily symptoms that are not caused by physical illness or injury
- thoughts of death or suicide, or suicide attempts

A depressive episode is diagnosed if five or more of these symptoms last most of the day, nearly every day, for a period of two weeks or longer.

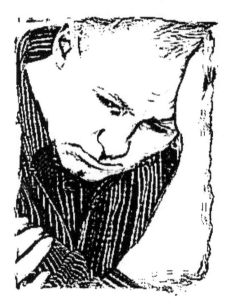

A mild to moderate level of mania is called hypomania. Hypomania may feel good to the person who experiences it and may even be associated with good functioning and enhanced productivity. Thus even when family and friends learn to recognise the mood swings as possible Bipolar Disorder, the person may deny that anything is wrong. Without proper treatment, however, hypomania can become severe mania in some people or can switch into depression.

Sometimes, severe episodes of mania or depression include symptoms of psychosis (or psychotic symptoms). Common psychotic symptoms are hallucinations (hearing, seeing or otherwise sensing the presence of things not actually there) and delusions (false, strongly held beliefs not influenced by logical reasoning or explained by a person's usual cultural concepts). Psychotic symptoms in Bipolar disorder tend to reflect the extreme mood state at the time. For example delusions of grandiosity, such as believing one is the President or has special powers or wealth, may occur during mania. Delusions of guilt or worthlessness, such as believing that one is ruined and penniless or has committed some terrible crime, may appear during depression. People with Bipolar Disorder who have these symptoms are sometimes incorrectly diagnosed as having Schizophrenia, another severe mental illness.

It may be helpful to think of the various mood states in Bipolar Disorder as a spectrum or continuous range. At one end is severe depression, above which is moderate depression and then mild low mood, which many people call "the blues" when it is short-lived but is termed "dysthymia" when it is chronic. Then there is normal or balanced mood, above which comes hypomania (mild to moderate mania), and then severe mania.

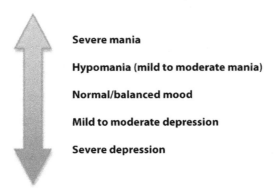

Severe mania

Hypomania (mild to moderate mania)

Normal/balanced mood

Mild to moderate depression

Severe depression

In some people however, symptoms of mania and depression may occur together in what is called a mixed bipolar state. Symptoms of a mixed state often include agitation, trouble sleeping, significant change in appetite, psychosis and suicidal thinking. A person may have a very sad, hopeless mood while at the same time feeling extremely energised.

Bipolar disorder may appear to be a problem other than mental illness—for instance, alcohol or drug abuse, poor school or work performance, or strained interpersonal relationships. Such problems in fact may be signs of an underlying mood disorder.

DIAGNOSIS OF BIPOLAR DISORDER

Like other mental illnesses, Bipolar disorder cannot yet be identified physiologically—for example, through a blood test or a brain scan. Therefore, a diagnosis of Bipolar Disorder is made on the basis of symptoms, course of illness, and when available, family history. The diagnostic criteria for bipolar disorder are described in the Diagnostic and Statistical Manual for Mental Disorders, fourth edition (DSM-IV).3

Descriptions offered by people with Bipolar Disorder give valuable insights into the various mood states associated with the illness:-

Depression: I doubt completely my ability to do anything well. It seems as though my mind has slowed down and burned out to the point of being virtually useless.... I am haunted... with the total, the desperate hopelessness of it all....

Others say, "It's only temporary, it will pass, you will get over it," but of course they haven't any idea of how I feel, although they are certain they do. If I can't feel, move, think or care, then what on earth is the point?

Hypomania: At first when I'm high, it's tremendous... ideas are fast... like shooting stars you follow until brighter ones appear…. All shyness disappears, the right words and gestures are suddenly there… uninteresting people, things become intensely interesting. Sensuality is pervasive, the desire to seduce and be seduced is irresistible. You are infused with unbelievable feelings of ease, power, well-being, omnipotence, euphoria… you can do anything… but, somewhere this changes.

Mania: The fast ideas become too fast and there are far too many… overwhelming confusion replaces clarity… you stop keeping up with it—memory goes. Infectious humour ceases to amuse. Your friends become frightened…. everything is now against the grain… you are irritable, angry, frightened, uncontrollable and trapped.

Some people with Bipolar disorder become suicidal. Anyone who is thinking about committing suicide needs immediate attention, preferably from a mental health professional or a physician. Anyone who talks about suicide should be taken seriously. Risk for suicide appears to be higher earlier in the course of the illness. Therefore, recognising Bipolar Disorder early and learning how best to manage it may decrease the risk of death by suicide.

Signs and symptoms that may accompany suicidal feelings include:-

- talking about feeling suicidal or wanting to die
- feeling hopeless, that nothing will ever change or get better
- feeling helpless, that nothing one does makes any difference
- feeling like a burden to family and friends
- abusing alcohol or drugs
- putting affairs in order (e.g. organising finances or giving away possessions to prepare for one's death)
- writing a suicide note
- putting oneself in harm's way, or in situations where there is a danger of being killed

If you are feeling suicidal or know someone who is:-

- call a doctor or emergency services right away to get immediate help
- make sure you, or the suicidal person, are not left alone
- make sure that access is prevented to large amounts of medication, weapons or other items that could be used for self-harm

While some suicide attempts are carefully planned over time, others are impulsive acts that have not been well thought out. Therefore, the final point in the list above may be a valuable long-term strategy for people with Bipolar Disorder. Either way, it is important to understand that suicidal feelings and actions are symptoms of an illness that can be treated. With proper treatment, suicidal feelings can be overcome.

Episodes of mania and depression typically recur across the life span. Between episodes most people with Bipolar Disorder are free of symptoms. But as many as one third of people have some residual symptoms. A small percentage of people experience chronic unremitting symptoms despite treatment.

The classic form of the illness, which involves recurrent episodes of mania and depression, is called Bipolar I Disorder. Some people however, never develop severe mania but instead experience milder episodes of hypomania that alternate with depression. This form of the illness is called Bipolar II Disorder. When four or more episodes of illness occur within a twelve month period, a person is said to have Rapid-Cycling Bipolar Disorder. Some people experience multiple episodes within a single week, or even within a single day. Rapid cycling tends to develop later in the course of illness and is more common among women than among men.

People with Bipolar disorder can lead healthy and productive lives when the illness is effectively treated (see below—"How Is Bipolar Disorder Treated?"). Without treatment, however, the natural course of Bipolar disorder tends to worsen. Over time a person may suffer more frequent (more rapid-cycling) and more severe manic and depressive episodes than those experienced when the illness first appeared. But in most cases proper treatment can help reduce the frequency and severity of episodes and can help people with Bipolar Disorder maintain good quality of life.

Let's take a look at various treatment options, both mainstream and non-mainstream. We'll be discussing these later in the book.

As an addition to medication psychosocial treatments, including certain forms of psychotherapy (or talk therapy), are helpful in providing support, education and guidance to people with Bipolar Disorder and their families. Studies have shown that psychosocial interventions can lead to increased mood stability, fewer hospitalisations and improved functioning in several areas. A psychologist, social worker or counsellor typically provides these therapies and often works together with the psychiatrist to monitor a patient's progress. The number, frequency and type of sessions should be based on the treatment needs of each person.

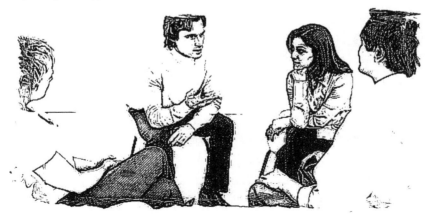

Psychosocial interventions commonly used for Bipolar disorder are Cognitive Behavioural Therapy (CBT), psychoeducation, family therapy and a newer technique, interpersonal and social rhythm therapy. NIMH researchers are studying how these interventions compare to one another when added to medication treatment for Bipolar Disorder.

Cognitive Behavioural Therapy helps people with Bipolar Disorder learn to change inappropriate or negative thought patterns and behaviours associated with the illness.

Psychoeducation involves teaching people with Bipolar disorder about the illness and its treatment, and how to recognise signs of relapse so that early intervention can be sought before a full-blown illness episode occurs. Psychoeducation also may be helpful for family members.

Family therapy uses strategies to reduce the level of distress within the family that may either contribute to or result from the ill person's symptoms.

Interpersonal and Social Rhythm Therapy helps people with Bipolar Disorder both to improve interpersonal relationships and to regularise their daily routines. Regular daily routines and sleep schedules may help protect against manic episodes. As with medication, it is important to follow the treatment plan for any psychosocial intervention to achieve the greatest benefit.

In situations where medication, psychosocial treatment and the combination of these interventions prove ineffective, or work too slowly to relieve severe symptoms such as psychosis or suicidal tendencies, Electroconvulsive Therapy (ECT) may be considered. ECT may also be considered to treat acute episodes when medical conditions, including pregnancy, make the use of medications too risky. ECT is a highly effective treatment for severe depressive, manic, and/or mixed episodes. The possibility of long-lasting memory problems, although a concern in the past, has been significantly reduced with modern ECT techniques. However the potential benefits and risks of ECT, and of available alternative interventions, should be carefully reviewed and discussed with individuals considering this treatment and, where appropriate, with family or friends.

Herbal or natural supplements, such as St. John's Wort (Hypericum Perforatum), have not been well studied, and little is known about their effects on Bipolar Disorder. Before trying herbal or natural supplements it is important to discuss them with your doctor. There is evidence that St. John's Wort can reduce the effectiveness of certain medications.

In addition, as with prescription antidepressants, St. John's Wort may cause a switch into mania in some individuals with Bipolar Disorder, especially if no mood stabiliser is being taken.

Omega-3 fatty acids found in fish oil are being studied to determine their usefulness, alone and when added to conventional medications, for long-term treatment of Bipolar Disorder.

It is important to note that even though episodes of mania and depression naturally come and go, it is important to understand that Bipolar Disorder is a long-term illness that currently has no cure. Staying on treatment even during well times, can help keep the disease under control and reduce the chance of having recurrent, worsening episodes.

Here is an image of our mood compass, a simple device that we will be introducing to you in the next chapter. This simple visual record will enable you to monitor the progress of your illness in a very straightforward and visual way, moreover one that will show you how the different aspects of your physiological and emotional characteristics interact with and influence one another. Filling in a mood compass should become a regular part of your recovery and therapy process. It will enable you to understand very readily when you are likely to experience highs and lows of mood, and very importantly how you dealt with these before.

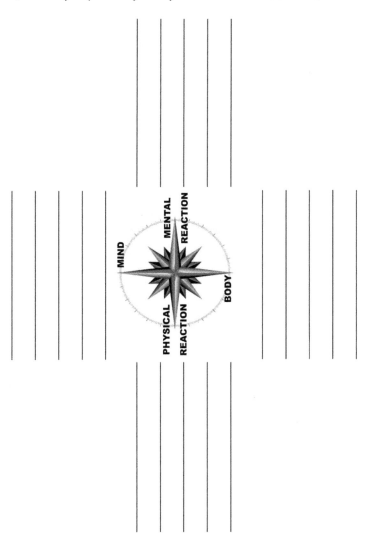

CHAPTER TWO

DO I HAVE BIPOLAR DISORDER OR IS IT ALL IN THE MIND?

"To confess ignorance is often wiser than to beat about the bush with a hypothetical diagnosis."

William Osler

The first step in getting treatment for Bipolar Disorder is getting a correct diagnosis. This can be a more difficult than it might seem because the symptoms of Bipolar can be similar at times to other major brain disorders, such as Schizophrenia or major depression. Because many regular family doctors may not be very familiar with Bipolar, it is important to see a therapist or psychiatrist who is experienced in the diagnosis and treatment of Bipolar or Schizophrenia. One way to do this is to contact a local support group that deals with brain disorders such as Schizophrenia and talk to the other members that already have experience with the local psychiatrists. As with most serious illnesses, it is important to get diagnosis and treatment as quickly as possible.

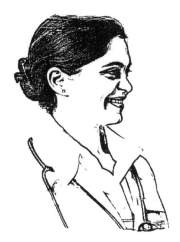 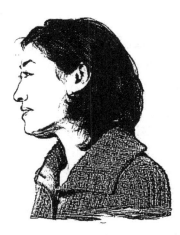

Unfortunately, there's no simple quick and easy test to diagnose people suspected of experiencing Bipolar Disorder. In fact, this ailment is not even a single disorder. Rather, it is a term used to describe a number of mood disorders that are identified by mania or manic episodes, bouts of depression and possibly psychotic episodes. One of or all the above can be present, making a simple and easy test for the disorder difficult to put together.

The act of seeing a psychiatrist or therapist can often cause much anxiety when really you just need to try to be in control and able to explain your problems as much as possible. The technique is actually very simple - it's all a matter of preparation.

Sit down a day or two before your appointment and make a list of everything you are feeling, with details about triggers and how your life is affected by each item.

For example:

- I have to walk to the other end of the store when babies are crying because I can't take the noise.
- I don't always believe people are who they say they are.
- I can get very angry, to the point of rage. (If there are patterns to things that trigger your anger, include them.)
- Several friends are angry at me because I have become inappropriately angry.
- I feel depressed frequently
- I feel very lonely and an extreme need for support. As a result I spend a lot of time crying.
- I can only get a few hours of sleep a night, sometimes none at all, or I am sleeping eighteen hours a day.

The key issue when listing these is to tell how they have impacted your life. DO NOT put labels on these feelings - let the doctor do that! Doctors often allow their patient's labels to block their own thought processes and sometimes allowing the patient to make the diagnosis. Again, you just want to list what you are feeling and how your life is affected.

I really recommend you take the time to do this.

When you break down the feelings, and how they are affecting your daily life, you paint a very clear picture for the doctor. You can't do that on the spot in a short visit when your brain is spinning and you don't know what to say first. So make the list. Then make three copies - two for yourself and one for the doctor. Leave one copy at home (it's just in case something happens to the copy you take for yourself) and take the other two with you. When you see the doctor, give them the list. You won't have to remember everything you wanted to tell them on the spot. You won't have to go away beating yourself up because you forgot to say something. You won't need to worry so much at all!

You are by no means alone in experiencing the alternate sensations of depression and manic activity that are a feature of Bipolar Disorder. It is increasingly common in today's society and causes a great deal of upset and distress to the sufferers and the people around them. Neither would you be alone if you were to put off seeing a doctor for as long as possible. It is quite normal to feel isolated, and possibly rejected, by other people, without fully understanding that the reason for this feeling is due to the progress of your illness rather than any personal fault. You may see a doctor and get a diagnosis of being Bipolar and refuse to believe it. Perhaps you feel that this kind of mental illness, previously known as Manic Depression, could not possibly describe the problems you are experiencing. All of these reactions to suffering the symptoms of Bipolar Disorder are quite normal. They do also have one other thing in common - they are unanimously incorrect. With any personal difficulty or illness you may be suffering, the first and most important step is to have that problem diagnosed professionally. Then face up to the process of dealing with it, either by finding a cure or by finding means to mitigate the symptoms. Hopefully at the very least mitigate the very worst of what you are suffering.

The diagnosis itself is unlikely to entirely satisfy you, even after you have accepted the fact of your disorder being Bipolar. You may feel victimised, perhaps even feel that the accusing finger of society is pointing at you as somebody suffering from a serious mental illness. You may feel that the whole question of a diagnosis of bipolar Disorder is unfair and unjust, almost society inflicting new punishment at a time when you simply feel "not yourself". However, it is important that you understand that clinical professionals, therapists, psychologists and psychiatrists do need to have standardised diagnostic tools to work with. Hopefully they will have a sufficiently good "bedside manner" to explain to you the necessity for using standardised tools and diagnostic procedures so that they can make an effective treatment plan for your illness. Equally they should be able to point out that using standardised diagnostic techniques is not intended to be impersonal. It is just an effort to be as accurate as possible in the patient's own best interests.

Following the diagnosis your therapist will then use their best efforts to help you deal with further episodes. There are a number of questions that you will have.

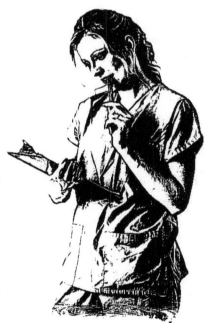

- How often are you likely to experience the return of the illness?
- Can it be cured?
- Will there be intervals between the opposite extremes of manic and oppressive behaviour when you experience no symptoms?

Following a thorough diagnosis these are hopefully the kinds of questions that a therapist will be able to answer for you, at least where an answer is possible.

The DSM IV definitions of bipolar disorder are as follows:

Bipolar I Disorder--Diagnostic Features (DSM-IV, p. 350)

The essential feature of Bipolar I Disorder is a clinical course that is characterized by the occurrence of one or more Manic Episodes or Mixed Episodes. Often individuals have also had one or more Major Depressive Episodes. Episodes of Substance-Induced Mood Disorder (due to the direct effects of a medication, or other somatic treatments for depression, a drug of abuse, or toxin exposure) or of Mood Disorder Due to a General Medical Condition do not count toward a diagnosis of Bipolar I Disorder. In addition, the episodes are not better accounted for by Schizoaffective Disorder and are not superimposed on Schizophrenia, Schizophreniform Disorder, Delusional Disorder, or Psychotic Disorder Not Otherwise Specified....

Bipolar II Disorder--Diagnostic Features (DSM-IV, p. 359)

The essential feature of Bipolar II Disorder is a clinical course that is characterized by the occurrence of one or more Major Depressive Episodes accompanied by at least one Hypomanic Episode. Hypomanic Episodes should not be confused with the several days of euthymia that may follow remission of a Major Depressive Episode. Episodes of Substance- Induced Mood Disorder (due to the direct effects of a medication, or other somatic treatments for depression, a drug of abuse, or toxin exposure) or of Mood Disorder Due to a General Medical Condition do not count toward a diagnosis of Bipolar I Disorder. In addition, the episodes are not better accounted for by Schizoaffective Disorder and are not superimposed on Schizophrenia, Schizophreniform Disorder, Delusional Disorder, or Psychotic Disorder Not Otherwise Specified.

The illness of course has two distinct phases in the use of the term Bipolar. The phases are manic and depressive. Some typical symptoms during both phases are as follows:-

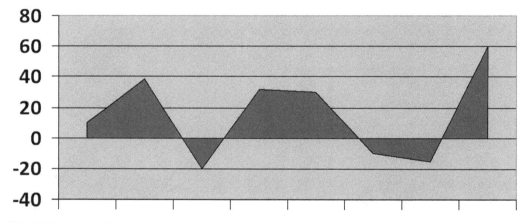

SIGNS OF A MANIC EPISODE/ MANIA

- agitation
- aggressive behaviour
- decreased need for sleep without fatigue
- denial that anything is wrong
- difficulty concentrating
- drug abuse (especially cocaine, alcohol and sleeping medications)
- exaggerated optimism
- excessively high or euphoric mood

- extreme irritability
- impulsiveness
- increased drive to perform or achieve goals
- increased physical and mental activity and energy
- increased restlessness
- increased sexual drive
- inflated self-esteem
- poor judgment
- provocative, intrusive, or aggressive behavior
- racing thoughts jumping from one idea to another
- risky behaviors
- shopping sprees
- talking very fast
- unrealistic beliefs in one's abilities and powers

SIGNS OF A DEPRESSIVE EPISODE / DEPRESSION

- chronic pain not caused by physical illness or injury
- decreased energy,
- difficulty concentrating, remembering, making decisions
- feeling fatigued or of being "slowed down"
- feelings of guilt, worthlessness, or helplessness
- feelings of hopelessness or pessimism
- indifference
- irritability, anger, worry, agitation, anxiety
- loss of energy, persistent lethargy
- loss of interest or pleasure in activities once enjoyed, including sex
- recurring thoughts of death or suicide, or suicide attempts
- restlessness
- sad, anxious, or empty mood
- significant changes in appetite
- sleeping too much, or difficulty sleeping
- social withdrawal
- weight loss or gain (unintentional)

The deep mood swings of Bipolar Disorder may last for weeks or months. Research suggests that Bipolar Disorder manifests a wide range of symptoms. The main characteristics of Bipolar Disorder are quick changes from mania to depression and back again. The periods of highs and lows are called "episodes". Mood episodes are intense. The feelings are strong and happen along with extreme changes in behaviour and energy levels. The signs and symptoms of manic episodes and depressive episodes are as follows.

CRITERIA FOR A MAJOR DEPRESSIVE EPISODE ARE:-

Five or more of the following symptoms have been present during the same two week period and represent a change from previous functioning. At least one of the symptoms is either number one or two.

1. Depressed mood most of the day, nearly every day, as indicated by either subjective report (e.g., feels sad or empty) or observation made by others (e.g., appears tearful). Note: In children and adolescents, can be irritable mood.

2. Markedly diminished interest or pleasure in all, or almost all, activities most of the day, nearly every day (as indicated by either subjective account or observation made by others).

3. Significant weight loss when not dieting or weight gain (e.g., a change of more than 5% of body weight in a month), or decrease or increase in appetite nearly every day. Note: In children, consider failure to make expected weight gains.

4. Insomnia or Hypersomnia nearly every day.

5. Psychomotor agitation or retardation nearly every day (observable by others, not merely subjective feelings of restlessness or being slowed down).

6. Fatigue or loss of energy nearly every day.

7. Feelings of worthlessness or excessive or inappropriate guilt (which may be delusional) nearly every day (not merely self-reproach or guilt about being sick).

8. Diminished ability to think or concentrate, or indecisiveness, nearly every day (either by subjective account or as observed by others).

9. Recurrent thoughts of death (not just fear of dying), recurrent suicidal ideation without a specific plan, or a suicide attempt or a specific plan for committing suicide.

CRITERIA FOR A MIXED EPISODE DSM-IV-TR

1. The criteria are met both for a Manic Episode and for a Major Depressive Episode (except for duration) nearly every day during at least a 1 week period.

2. The mood disturbance is sufficiently severe to cause marked impairment in occupational functioning or in usual social activities or relationships with others, or to necessitate hospitalisation to prevent harm to self or others, or there are psychotic features.

3. The symptoms are not due to the direct physiological effects of a substance (e.g., an illicit drug, a medication, or other treatment) or a general medical condition

CRITERIA FOR A MANIC EPISODE DSM-IV-TR

A distinct period of abnormally and persistently elevated, expansive or irritable mood, lasting at least one week (or any duration if hospitalisation is necessary).

During the period of mood disturbance, three (or more) of the following symptoms have persisted (four if the mood is only irritable) and have been present to a significant degree:

1. Inflated self-esteem or grandiosity, potentially including grandiose delusions.
2. Decreased need for sleep (e.g., feels rested after only three hours of sleep) or persistent difficulty falling asleep
3. More talkative than usual or pressure to keep talking.
4. Fight of ideas or subjective experience that thoughts are racing.
5. Distractibility (i.e., attention too easily drawn to unimportant or irrelevant external stimuli)
6. Increase in goal-directed activity (either socially, at work or school, or sexually) or psychomotor agitation.
7. Excessive involvement in pleasurable activities that have a high potential for painful consequences (e.g., engaging in unrestrained buying sprees, sexual indiscretions, or foolish business investments).

A study published last year suggested that Bipolar Disorder, formerly Manic-Depressive Disorder or Manic-Depression, may be over diagnosed in people seeking mental health care. Now new findings shed light on which disorders many of these patients actually have.

In a 2008 study, researchers at Brown University School of Medicine found that of 145 adults who said they had been diagnosed with Bipolar Disorder, 82 (57%) turned out not to have the condition when given a comprehensive diagnostic interview. In a later study, published in the Journal of Clinical Psychiatry, the researchers used similar standardised interviews to find out which disorders those 82 patients might have.

Overall, they found, nearly half had major depression or borderline Personality Disorder. A personality disorder marked by a long-standing pattern of instability in interpersonal relationships, behaviour, mood and self-image that can interfere with social or occupational functioning or cause extreme, Post-Traumatic Stress Disorder PTSD (mental disorder that follows an occurrence of extreme psychological stress, such as that encountered in war or resulting from violence, childhood abuse, sexual abuse or a serious accident).

When the researchers then compared the patients with 528 other psychiatric patients who had never been diagnosed with Bipolar Disorder, they found that those in the former group were nearly four times more likely to have Borderline Personality Disorder. They were also 70% more likely to have major depression and twice as likely to have PTSD.

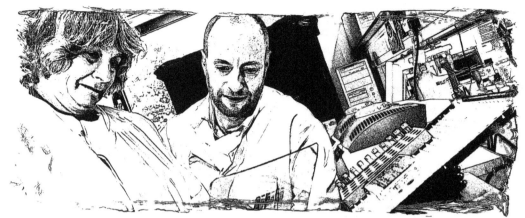

Some other diagnoses were less common, but still seen at elevated rates among the patients previously diagnosed with bipolar Disorder. These included Antisocial Personality Disorder (a personality disorder characterised by chronic antisocial behavior and violation of the law and the rights of others) and Impulse-Control Disorder.

Over diagnosis of Bipolar Disorder is of concern, in part, because it is typically treated with mood-stabilising drugs that can have side effects. These include effects on the kidneys, liver and metabolic and immune systems. Bipolar Disorder shares certain characteristics with some other psychiatric conditions. Borderline Personality Disorder for instance is marked by unstable mood, impulsive behaviour and problems maintaining relationships with other people.

Doctors suspect that some therapists are over diagnosing Bipolar Disorder because, unlike certain other causes of mood disturbance, it does have effective drug therapies. There are no medications approved specifically for treating Borderline Personality Disorder, but research suggests that some forms of "talk therapy" are effective.

Bipolar Disorder has not currently been cured but it can be managed. It might be influencing clinicians, who are unsure whether or not a patient has Bipolar Disorder or Borderline Personality Disorder, to err on the side of diagnosing the disorder that is responsive to medication.

Here is a useful screening quiz that you can try filling in to assess the likelihood of your suffering from Bipolar Disorder:

1. At times I am much more talkative or speak much faster than usual.

    Not at all

    Just a little

    Somewhat

    Moderately

    Quite a lot

    Very much

2. There have been times when I was much more active or did many more things than usual.

    Not at all

    Just a little

    Somewhat

    Moderately

    Quite a lot

    Very much

3. I get into moods where I feel very speeded up or irritable.

    Not at all

    Just a little

    Somewhat

    Moderately

    Quite a lot

    Very much

4. There have been times when I have felt both high (elated) and low (depressed) at the same time.

Not at all

Just a little

Somewhat

Moderately

Quite a lot

Very much

5. At times I have been much more interested in sex than usual.

Not at all

Just a little

Somewhat

Moderately

Quite a lot

Very much

6. My self-confidence ranges from great self-doubt to equally great overconfidence.

Not at all

Just a little

Somewhat

Moderately

Quite a lot

Very much

7. There have been GREAT variations in the quantity or quality of my work.

Not at all

Just a little

Somewhat

Moderately

Quite a lot

Very much

8. For no apparent reason I sometimes have been VERY angry or hostile.

Not at all

Just a little

Somewhat

Moderately

Quite a lot

Very much

9. I have periods of mental dullness and other periods of very creative thinking.

Not at all

Just a little

Somewhat

Moderately

Quite a lot

Very much

10. At times I am greatly interested in being with people and at other times I just want to be left alone with my thoughts.

Not at all

Just a little

Somewhat

Moderately

Quite a lot

Very much

11. I have had periods of great optimism and other periods of equally great pessimism.

Not at all

Just a little

Somewhat

Moderately

Quite a lot

Very much

12. I have had periods of tearfulness and crying and other times when I laugh and joke excessively.

Not at all

Just a little

Somewhat

Moderately

Quite a lot

Very much

You will notice that there are six alternative answers for each of the twelve questions, score one for the first answer, two the second answer and up to six for the last answer. The possible scores can range from twelve (which would be a person with virtually no likelihood whatsoever of suffering from Bipolar Disorder), to seventy two (which would suggest a person with very severe symptoms indeed).

When you take this test use your own judgement as to how severe you feel it shows that your symptoms to be. In general, any score that is higher than the middle ranking of thirty six indicates that the person should seek some kind of advice from a medical professional.

Here is a useful table that shows clearly the various symptoms, treatments and outcomes of bipolar disorder which will give you a very good idea of exactly what is involved.

BIPOLAR SYNOPSIS

Bipolar I Disorder is one of the most severe forms of mental illness and is characterized by recurrent episodes of mania and (more often) depression. The condition has a high rate of recurrence and if untreated, it has an approximately 15% risk of death by suicide. It is the third leading cause of death among people aged 15-24 years, and is the 6th leading cause of disability (lost years of healthy life) for people aged 15-44 years in the developed world.

CAUSATION

Bipolar I Disorder is a life-long disease and runs in families but has a complex mode of inheritance. Family, twin and adoption studies suggest genetic factors. The concordance rate for monozygotic (identical) twins is 43%; whereas it is only 6% for dizygotic (nonidentical) twins. About half of all patients with Bipolar I Disorder have one parent who also has a mood disorder, usually Major Depressive Disorder. If one parent has Bipolar I Disorder, the child will have a 25% chance of developing a mood disorder (about half of these will have Bipolar I or II Disorder, while the other half will have Major Depressive Disorder). If both parents have Bipolar I Disorder, the child has a 50%-75% chance of developing a mood disorder. First-degree biological relatives of individuals with Bipolar I Disorder have elevated rates of Bipolar I Disorder (4%-24%), Bipolar II Disorder (1%-5%), and Major Depressive Disorder (4%-24%).

The finding that the concordance rate for monozygotic twins isn't 100% suggests that environmental or psychological factors likely play a role in causation. Certain environmental factors (e.g., antidepressant medication, antipsychotic medication, electroconvulsive therapy, stimulants) or certain illnesses (e.g., multiple sclerosis, brain tumor, hyperthyroidism) can trigger mania. Mania can be triggered by giving birth, sleep deprivation, and major stressful life events.

SYMPTOMS

In adults, mania is usually episodic with an elevation of mood and increased energy and activity. In children, mania is commonly chronic rather than episodic, and usually presents in mixed states with irritability, anxiety and depression. In adults and children, during depression there is lowering of mood and decreased energy and activity. During a mixed episode both mania and depression can occur on the same day.

COMORBIDITY

Comorbidity is the rule, not the exception, in bipolar disorder. The most common mental disorders that co-occur with bipolar disorder are anxiety, substance use, and conduct disorders. Disorders of eating, sexual behavior, attention-deficit/hyperactivity, and impulse control, as well as autism spectrum disorders and Tourette's disorder, co-occur with bipolar disorder. The most common general medical comorbidities are migraine, thyroid illness, obesity, type II diabetes, and cardiovascular disease.

ASSOCIATED MENTAL DISORDERS

Bipolar I Disorder is often associated with: alcoholism, drug addiction, Anorexia Nervosa, Bulimia Nervosa, Attention-Deficit Hyperactivity Disorder, Panic Disorder, and Social Phobia.

DIAGNOSTIC TESTS

There are no diagnostic laboratory tests for Bipolar I Disorder. Thus diagnosis is arrived at by using standardized diagnostic criteria to rate the patient's behavior. Onset of mania after age 40 could signify that the mania may be due to a general medical condition or substance use. Current or past hypothyroidism (or even mild thyroid hypofunction) may be associated with Rapid Cycling. Hyperthyroidism may precipitate or worsen mania in individuals with a preexisting Mood Disorder. However, hyperthyroidism in individuals without preexisting Mood Disorder does not typically cause manic symptoms.

DIFFERENTIAL DIAGNOSIS

Bipolar I Disorder must be distinguished from:

- Mood Disorder Due to a General Medical Condition (e.g., due to multiple sclerosis, stroke, hypothyroidism, or brain tumor)
- Substance-Induced Mood Disorder (e.g., due to drug abuse, antidepressant medication, or electroconvulsive therapy)
- Other Mood Disorders (e.g., Major Depressive Disorder; Dysthymia; Bipolar II Disorder; Cyclothymic Disorder)
- Psychotic Disorders (e.g., Schizoaffective Disorder, Schizophrenia, or Delusional Disorder)
- Since this disorder may be associated with hyperactivity, recklessness, impulsivity, and antisocial behavior; the diagnosis of Bipolar I Disorder must be carefully differentiated from Attention Deficit Hyperactivity Disorder, Conduct Disorder, Antisocial Personality Disorder, and Borderline Personality Disorder Pathophysiology

The pathophysiology of Bipolar I Disorder is poorly understood. However, a variety of imaging studies suggests the involvement of structural abnormalities in the amygdala, basal ganglia and prefrontal cortex. Research is now showing that this disorder is associated with abnormal brain levels of serotonin, norepinephrine, and dopamine.

PREVALENCE

Bipolar I Disorder affects both sexes equally in all age groups and its worldwide prevalence is approximately 3-5%. It can even present in preschoolers. There are no significant differences among racial groups in the prevalence of this disorder.

COURSE

The first episode may occur at any age from childhood to old age. The average age at onset is 21. More than 90% of individuals who have a single Manic Episode go on to have future episodes. Untreated patients with Bipolar I Disorder typically have 8 to 10 episodes of mania and depression in their lifetime. Often 5 years or more may elapse between the first and second episode, but thereafter the episodes become more frequent and more severe.

There is significant symptom reduction between episodes, but 25% of patients continue to display mood instability or mild depression. As many as 60% of patients experience chronic interpersonal or occupational difficulties between acute episodes. Bipolar I Disorder may develop psychotic symptoms. The psychotic symptoms in Bipolar I Disorder only occur during severe manic, mixed or depressive episodes. In contrast, the psychotic symptoms in Schizophrenia can occur when there is no mania or depression. Poor recovery is more common after psychosis.

Manic episodes usually begin abruptly and last for between 2 weeks and 4-5 months (median duration about 4 months). Depressive episodes tend to last longer (median length about 6 months), though rarely for more than a year, except in the elderly.

TREATMENT AND OUTCOME

The usual treatment for Bipolar I Disorder is lifelong therapy with a mood-stabilizer (either lithium, carbamazepine, or divalproex / valproic acid) often in combination with an antipsychotic medication. Usually treatment results in a dramatic decrease in suffering, and causes an 8-fold reduction in suicide risk. In mania, an antipsychotic medication and/or a benzodiazepine medication is often added to the mood-stabilizer. In depression, quetiapine, olanzapine, or lamotrigine is often added to the mood-stabilizer. Alternatively, in depression, the mood-stabilizer can be switched to another mood-stabilizer, or two mood-stabilizers can be used together. Sometimes, in depression, antidepressant medication is used. Since antidepressant medication can trigger mania, antidepressant medication should always be combined with a mood-stablizer or antipsychotic medication to prevent mania.

Research has shown that the most effective treatment is a combination of supportive psychotherapy, psychoeducation, and the use of a mood-stabilizer (often combined with an antipsychotic medication). There is no research showing that any form of psychotherapy is an effective substitute for medication. Likewise there is no research showing that any "health food store nutritional supplement" (e.g., vitamin, amino acid) is effective for Bipolar I Disorder.

Since a Manic Episode can quickly escalate and destroy a patient's career or reputation, a therapist must be prepared to hospitalize out-of-control manic patients before they "lose everything". Likewise, severely depressed, suicidal bipolar patients often require hospitalization to save their lives.

Although the medication therapy for Bipolar I Disorder usually must be lifelong, the majority of bipolar patients are noncompliant and stop their medication after one year. At 4-year follow-up of bipolar patients, 41% have a good overall outcome and 4% have died. Women with bipolar disorder lose, on average, 9 years in life expectancy, 14 years of lost productivity and 12 years of normal health

BEST RECOVERIES

The best recoveries are achieved when individuals with Bipolar I Disorder:

1. Get the correct diagnosis (since many are misdiagnosed as having schizophrenia or "just borderline personality")

2. Get effective treatment and faithfully stay on it for a lifetime (most individuals require the combination of a mood-stabilizer plus an antipsychotic medication)

3. Adopt a healthy lifestyle (regular sleep and exercise; no alcohol or drug abuse; low stress)

4. Regularly see a supportive physician who is knowledgeable about the psychiatric management of this disorder

5. Learn which symptoms predict the return of this illness, and what additional "rescue" medication should be taken

6. Learn to trust the warnings given by family and friends when they see early signs of relapse

7. Learn as much as possible about this illness from therapists, the Internet, books, or self-help groups

TREATMENT FOR DEPRESSIVE EPISODE

Proven (Better Than Placebo) Treatments for Bipolar Depression

- Lithium and anticonvulsants prevent suicide [1, 2, 3, 4]
- Lithium (for prevention of future depression and suicide)
- Carbamazepine (for prevention of future depression)
- Lamotrigine (for depression)
- Olanzapine (for suicidal ideation in bipolar I manic or mixed-episode patients)
- Quetiapine (for depression)
- Fluoxetine (for depression)
- Imipramine (for depression but not prevention of future depression)
- Tranylcypromine (for depression)

Promising (But Unproven) Treatments for Bipolar Depression

- Amitriptyline (with mood-stabilizer)
- Cognitive Therapy (with mood-stabilizer)
- Electroconvulsive Therapy (no placebo-controlled trials)
- Family Psychoeducation (with mood-stabilizer)
- Group Psychoeducation (with mood-stabilizer)
- L-Sulpiride (with mood-stabilizer)
- Moclobemide (with mood-stabilizer)

- Paroxetine (with mood-stabilizer)
- Psychotherapy (with mood-stabilizer)
- Venlafaxine (with mood-stabilizer)

Ineffective Treatments for Depression

- No additional benefit of adding antidepressant medication to a mood stabilizer
- Do certain medications for Bipolar Disorder increase suicidal risk? [1, 2, 3, 4, 5, 6, 7]

Illness Course for Depression

- Bipolar Disorder and severe Major Depressive Disorder are episodic, life-long illnesses that need life-long prophylactic treatment
- Untreated depressive episodes usually last 11 weeks
- Usually there are multiple episodes of depression if untreated
- Suicide rate for bipolar patients is 15-22 times the national average
- Suicide rate in first year off lithium therapy is 20 times the rate when on lithium

TREATMENT FOR DEPRESSIVE EPISODE

Proven (Better Than Placebo)Treatments for Mania

- Monotherapy (treatment with just one medication) for Bipolar Disorder is usually inadequate, and most patients require a combination of a mood-stabilizer and antipsychotic medication
- Lithium (for mania & prevention of future mania (59% success rate), but increases risk of diabetes insipidus and hypothyroidism)
- Carbamazepine (for mania & prevention of future mania)
- Divalproex sodium (for mania but not prevention of future mania, but increases risk of polycystic ovaries and hyperinsulinemia)
- No difference between in generic valproic acid and divalproex sodium in hospitalization
- Olanzapine (for mania but increases risk of weight gain & diabetes)
- Olanzapine (for suicidal ideation in bipolar I manic or mixed episodes)
- Quetiapine (for mania)
- Risperidone (for mania)
- Haloperidol (for mania)
- Caution: is the increased use of atypical antipsychotic medication (e.g., olanzapine) causing an increased risk of stroke, heart disease and hypertension?

Promising (But Unproven) Treatments for Mania

- Clozapine (but increases risk of diabetes and agranulocytosis)
- Electroconvulsive Therapy
- Lamotrigine (for prevention of future rapid-cycling)
- Phenytoin (with neuroleptic for mania}

Ineffective Treatments for Mania

- Gabapentin
- Verapamil
- Topiramate monotherapy or adjunctive therapy with Topiramate (and has serious side-effects)

Illness Course for Mania

- Untreated pure manic episodes usually last 6 weeks
- Untreated mixed (manic+depressive) episodes usually last 17 weeks
- Usually there are multiple episodes of mania if untreated
- Mania usually returns 5 months after stopping lithium therapy
- Within 2-4 years of first lifetime hospitalization for mania, 43% achieved functional recovery, and 57% switched or had new illness episodes

THE MOOD COMPASS

We now plan to introduce you to the concept of the Mood Compass. Clearly you have taken a giant leap to resolving your problems by accepting that you have a disorder that you need to come to grips with, either by yourself, with your physician or ideally in the company with other people who have considerable experience of dealing with this disorder.

With this acceptance you can now begin to look at the mood swings that occur to you from a different perspective. They are no longer the enemy, some dark amorphous mass that threatens to destroy your whole life. You are no longer the victim, but an active participant in the process of overcoming your disorder and once again living a happy, balanced and fulfilled life. It is very important that you chart a record of your progress, and in later chapters we will be introducing a range of different tools that will help you to achieve exactly this. To begin with, look at the Mood Compass, which like its namesake is a four pointed device has correlations to the differences in your mood.

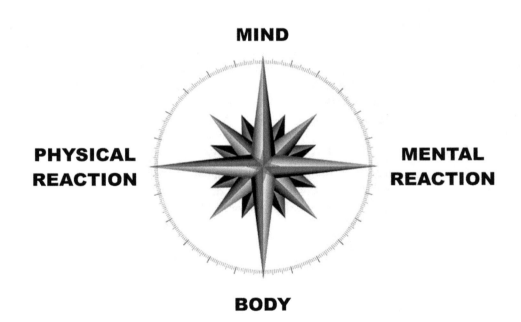

Think of the points of the compass - north, south, east and west. In a similar way we have devised a four point model to illustrate the complex relationships that together form a person's mental health. We will call this our 'mood compass'.

- Instead of North, think of the mind. The mind is that complex hub of physical and emotional influences. A very common characteristic of the mind that causes people to seek help from therapists is low self esteem.
- For South, we need to look at the model of the physical body, which in adversity will display such symptoms as chronic illness, acute illness, allergies and a range of symptoms ranging from a cut finger to severe heart problems.
- To the West of our compass style diagram we have identified physical reactions to a range of stimuli. These could be headaches, aches and pains, stiffness and soreness and occasionally more severe difficulties such as ME.
- Lastly to the East of our compass we can look at mental reactions to stimuli. These reactions are the kinds of things that will result in changes of mood. In the case of people seeking therapy these changes of mood will almost certainly be very severe indeed, at least in so far as the patient is concerned.

Sarah was a postgraduate student at a major university, studying social work. She had begun to experience extreme swings in her behaviour, whereby she often went for several days at the time without sleep. She was causing a great deal of concern and alarm within her fellow students in the university hall where she resided, frequently banging their doors and trying to engage them in conversation in the early hours of the morning. It was almost as if she was taking some kind of drug to enhance her energy levels such as amphetamines or cocaine. Indeed, this was the first concern of her colleagues when her behaviour became so extreme.

After several days of this manic behaviour she then seems to disappear for two or three days. It afterwards emerged that she was sleeping a great deal during the depressive phase of her illness. When she did appear in company she was very withdrawn and miserable, as if she had a tremendous weight on her mind. After two or three days of depressive behaviour she would then swing into the manic phase and begin all over again causing mayhem at all hours of the day and night, especially at night when of course most people are happily asleep. Her behaviour came so excessive that she was eventually persuaded to seek psychiatric help and offered drugs to control her disorder. Initially it she took a course of drugs and found that her mood swings did moderate and she was able to live a more normal life, in this case continuing with her postgraduate studies. She did, however, worry about the long-term side effects of taking drugs to control her disorder.

Sarah filled in a Mood Compass, and the result was quite startling. She had not realised quite how extreme her moods were, and how enormous the swing between manic behaviour to the depressive behaviour was occurring. This was very encouraging, for she had taken the first step in being able to monitor her disorder and so be able to control it, at least in its more severe state at the outset. Because of the depth and severity of the disorder she elected to fill in a Mood Compass on a daily basis so that she had a visual reminder of exactly what she was going through, how she felt and how frequently it occurred.

At the end of Chapter 2 we would like you to become familiar with the Mood Compass. Make several copies of the Mood Compass with lines above and below and to either side for you to fill in with your own feelings and symptoms. It would be most useful if you were able to scan this into a computer and therefore print copies as and when you wanted them. Otherwise, you can use of photocopying service to make copies or even draw them yourself if you are so inclined. Keep your completed charts in a ring binder, with the most current sheet at the top. So that at any stage you can look back and monitor the progress of your mood swings.

Lastly, remember that Bipolar Disorder is an illness like any other illness. There is nothing to be achieved by attempting to keep it to yourself. On the contrary, one of the major problems facing Bipolar sufferers is that of isolation. If you are able to talk as calmly unreasonably as possible to your friends, family and co-workers about the way you feel it will help them to understand and accept exactly what kind of a battle you are facing. You should be proud of the steps you are taking to deal with and beat disorder.

Never feel shame, who knows about your illness!

The next person that you exchange a few words with about Bipolar Disorder could be a sufferer themselves, or have a close family member who may well be a sufferer. In this way not only will you help yourself to lose a great deal of your isolation, you may well help another sufferer to get more understanding of their own condition and on their own path to recovery.

One prominent Bipolar Disorder sufferer, who happened to be a well-known TV presenter, had this to say:

> "People who don't know what depression is, who say it's self-indulgence sound callous, but it's not callousness born of indifference. I think it's callousness born of ignorance. That kind of ignorance we've got to get rid of, and little by little 1 suppose, we will. You say to them, "It's a pity you don't know. I'm sure that if you knew, not only wouldn't you say that, you'd try to help in one way or another".

For myself and those who participate in the documentaries, it is empowering to speak out about mental illness. It helps provide validation, hope and the means to recover. Not to speak out is to live a lie, in the closet. By speaking out about your own experiences, it empowers all of us, and helps break down stigma. It is the most powerful action any of us can take. Add your voice and tell your story."

MENTAL REACTION

MIND

PHYSICAL REACTION

BODY

CHAPTER THREE

TO BE OR NOT BE BIPOLAR

"There is no greater mistake than the hasty conclusion that opinions are worthless because they are badly argued"

Thomas Henry Huxley

A question we are frequently asked is:-

"Do you really think I am Bipolar? That's impossible, I have always had periods of intense activity, then I get tired and of course I need time to recover. That's just part of life."

In this chapter we intend to describe an exhaustive list of conditions that may indicate a reasonable diagnosis of Bipolar Disorder, and equally importantly a long list of conditions that are frequently misdiagnosed as Bipolar Disorder. There is little doubt that people often suffer considerable anxiety when they exhibit signs of altered behaviour. The only way to deal with this anxiety of course is to form an accurate diagnosis as quickly and as professionally as possible. What we aim to do here is to give you the tools to enable you to understand more what is involved and what is not involved. In this way you will be equipped to make the correct choices and decisions to go forward with your condition, and hopefully to mitigate the symptoms or even find a course of treatment that causes them to disappear altogether.

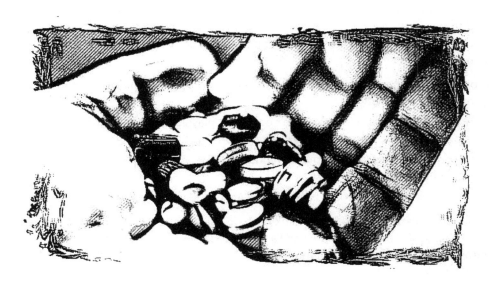

Here is a typical story from one sufferer, were they Bipolar or not?

>'To tell the truth - I'm not sure I am bipolar.
>
>I have been feeling more energetic the last couple of weeks, but that might not be due to being without a mood stabiliser. I have been off Depakote for several weeks now, and have been feeling better without it in some ways - less draggy.
>
>My current medication is 150 mg of Wellbutrin SR in the morning, at bedtime 50 mg Zoloft, 2.5 mg Zyprexa (for sleep) and 20 mg Zocor (for cholesterol). Decreasing the amount of Wellbutrin has taken care of the hot flushes. Now the main problem is the persistent bloating in my hands, which is driving me batty. To see whether Wellbutrin is the culprit here, we are going to cut the dosage down to 100 mg - but I have almost a full bottle of Wellbutrin SR 150s, and I hate like hell not to use them up. Prescriptions aren't free, after all!
>
>When I think that this whole carnival-ride-from-hell started because I wanted to lose the weight I had gained from Prozac and quitting smoking, without going into depression - I could cry. And I still have not lost any weight - in spite of all the walking I did over the summer, I've gained. Why does it have to be so complicated?
>
>Reading back over what I've written during the past five months, I don't know whether to call my experience a roller-coaster, an out-of-control carousel - maybe a Tilt-A-Whirl is closest. I've spun around in small circles while going round in a larger high-low circle at the same time.
>
>It's the pits. But I've been in blacker pits before.
>
>Five years and a few months ago, I was coming home from work each day, sitting down, and staring at the television all evening, blank-eyed. The room got messy around me, and I didn't care. I'd make a casserole of some kind and eat some every night till it was gone, that was dinner.

Depression has always been there. Over the years I have come up with mind-games to get myself out of a chair and into activity:

- Put a record on (yes, a record; I don't own a CD player) and pick up the mess (I live in a perpetual state of chaos) until the record's over;
- Turn on the timer and clean for ten minutes; then read or watch TV for 20 minutes; then clean for another ten minutes;
- Start in one corner of a room and JUST CLEAN;

Housecleaning, you see, was all I could think of to do that was active, as opposed to passively sitting in a chair. (AND - this was before I had a computer! Now the mess is ten times worse.) The way I knew my depression was becoming dangerous, at that time, was that all the mind-games had stopped working.

Now, with my weight staying 45-50 pounds over where it needs to be, with my fingers feeling like sausages as I type, having no idea what more I can do to get rid of this excess weight - I have an uneasy sense that depression is just around the corner again. "

Is this person Bipolar ? One thing is for sure. They are clearly suffering from some form of simple depressive condition at the very least, possibly an element Bipolar illness. They are taking a cocktail of drugs for, amongst other things, conditions they are not even certain they suffer from. Without very close professional guidance, this is a certain road to disaster. Have you ever found yourself in this position, or do you find yourself in this position now? Quite simply, if you are not sure whether or not you have Bipolar Disorder you need professional help and advice to at least form an initial diagnosis and begin dealing with the problem. After all, a return to good health and the optimum quality of life for you is very important.

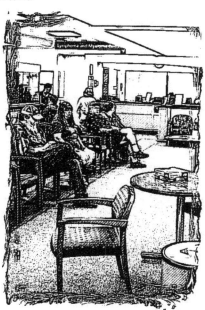

Bipolar Disorder is in fact somewhat less common than simple depression (i.e. clinical depression), and many people with Bipolar Disorder are misdiagnosed with depression. Part of the problem is that few patients are self-aware of their manic or euphoric episodes and only seek treatment during depressive times, and are then diagnosed with depression. However, depression is not the only possible misdiagnosis of Bipolar Disorder. Others include anxiety disorders, Borderline Personality Disorder and Schizophrenia. Unfortunately, many people with Bipolar Disorder are misdiagnosed for years.

The following conditions have been mentioned as possible alternative diagnoses to consider during the diagnostic process for Bipolar Disorder:-

Depression - Bipolar is often mistaken to be depression because treatment usually sought in the depressive phase, about half of people with Bipolar Disorder are misdiagnosed with Unipolar Depression.

- Clinical Depression
- Anxiety Disorder (type of Neurosis)
- Borderline Personality Disorder
- Antisocial Personality Disorder
- Schizophrenia
- Alcohol Abuse
- Drug Abuse
- Substance-induced Mood Disorder
- Substance Intoxication

- Schizoaffective Disorder
- Psychotic Disorder
- Dysthymia
- Cyclothymic Disorder
- Bipolar II Disorder
- Thyroid Disorder
- Bipolar Disorder
- Substance Abuse
- Hypomania
- Hyperthyroidism
- Medications
- Personality Disorder
- CNS Disease

Other illnesses for which Bipolar disorder is listed as a possible alternative diagnosis can include:-

- ADD
- Addiction
- Adult ADHD
- Attention Deficit Hyperactivity Disorder
- Borderline Personality Disorder
- Chronic Fatigue Syndrome
- Chronic Pelvic Pain
- Conduct Disorder
- Cyclothymic Disorder
- Delirium
- Depression
- Dissociative Identity Disorder
- Dysthymia/Seasonal Depression Disorder, PND
- Paraphilia
- Personality Disorders
- Social Phobia

Causes of Bipolar disorder may include these medical conditions:-

- People with an immediate family member with Bipolar Disorder are at higher risk.
- Genetic factors

- Environmental influence
- Childhood precursors

Rare Types of Bipolar Disorder:-

- Schizophrenic associated
- Schizoaffective disorders
- Reserpine induced depression
- Neurosyphilis
- Multiple Sclerosis
- Attention Deficit Hyperactivity Disorder
- Cylcothymic disorder

Commonly undiagnosed conditions in related areas may include:-

- Adult ADHD - Often remains undiagnosed through to adulthood.
- ADHD
- Alzheimer Disease
- Migraine
- Concentration Disorders
- Stroke
- Bipolar Disorder
- Schizophrenia
- Epilepsy

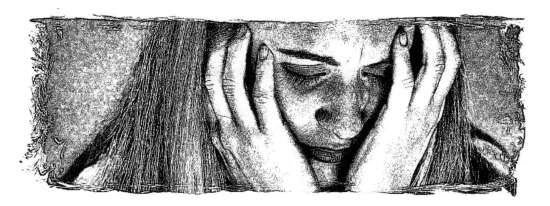

Bipolar Disorder may appear to be a problem other than mental illness. For instance alcohol or drug abuse, poor school or work performance, or strained interpersonal relationships. Such problems in fact may be signs of an underlying mood disorder. Bipolar Disorder in children and adolescents has been difficult to recognise and diagnose because it does not fit precisely the symptom criteria established for adults. Its symptoms can resemble or co-occur with those of ADHD and OCD. In addition, symptoms of Bipolar Disorder may be initially mistaken for normal emotions and behaviour of children and adolescents. But unlike normal mood changes, Bipolar Disorder significantly impairs functioning in school, with peers and at home with family.

Rare Epilepsy can cause a variety of severe emotional and depressive symptoms:. The book "Preventing Misdiagnosis of Women" reports on a case of a woman with severe personality and behavioural symptoms, and a diagnosis of Borderline Personality Disorder. She had extreme symptoms such as depression, cyclic moods, relationship problems, and many other emotional and neurological symptoms. After years of unsuccessful treatment, she was finally diagnosed with the rare Temporal Lobe Epilepsy, a form of epilepsy without seizures. Treatment for that disorder was highly effective and changed her life. Physical disorders are often hidden causes of depression. It is a common misdiagnosis to diagnose a psychological or psychiatric disorder, such as depression, when symptoms are actually caused by an underlying physical disorder. Some of the conditions that may cause depression-like symptoms include diabetes, thyroid disorders, chronic fatigue symptoms, endocrine disorders and many others. (see misdiagnosis of depression)

Underactive Thryoid may be misdiagnosed as depression. Hypothyroidism, underactive thyroid, is an endocrine gland disorder that is more common in women. It can mimic many diseases, including depression. The patient often has depressive type symptoms, and may also have other symptoms such as tingling fingers (peripheral neuropathy), hearing loss, headaches, and cold insensitivity. Common misdiagnoses of hypothyroidism include depression, dementia, Schizophrenia, or Bipolar disorder (especially Rapid-Cycling Bipolar Disorder). Cushing's Disease can be mistaken for depression. Cushing's disease (or similarly Cushing's Syndrome) is a possible misdiagnosis for a person diagnosed with depression. It is an endocrine disorder with many depressive-like characteristics, but also some physical symptoms. Cushing's Disease may also have schizophrenia-like symptoms such as paranoia and delusions, leading to a misdiagnosis of Schizophrenia. Manic or euphoria type symptoms are also possible, with a misdiagnosis of Bipolar Disorder.

Another uncommon endocrine disorder that can be misdiagnosed as depression is Hypocalcemia (low blood calcium), which is usually due to a disorder of the parathyroid gland called "hypoparathyroidism". This condition has many depressive symptoms, irritability, fatigue and others. A complex partial seizure disorder, such as Temporal lobe Epilepsy can be misdiagnosed as various conditions. Some of the possible misdiagnoses include depression, Bipolar Disorder, Schizophrenia, Borderline Personality Disorder, Multiple Personality Disorder, Somatization Disorder, Hypochondria, an anxiety disorder, sexuality disorders, hysteria and fatigue.

The early stages of Multiple Sclerosis may cause various general feelings of wellness, happiness, euphoria or manic-type symptoms in some patients. These symptoms may lead to a misdiagnosis of Bipolar Disorder (manic-depressive disorder), Hypomania, Cyclothymia, histrionic Personality Disorder or similar disorders. Other patients may show depressive symptoms as part of Multiple Sclerosis and risk a misdiagnosis of depression (i.e. Non-Bipolar Unipolar Depression). Other possible misdiagnoses of Multiple Sclerosis include Somatization Disorder, Conversion Disorder, neurotic disorders or other psychological disorders.

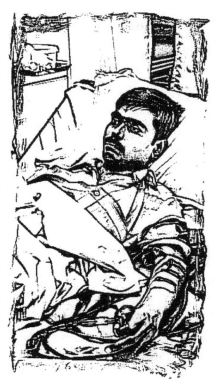

Lupus is often misdiagnosed as other conditions. Systemic Lupus Erythematosus (SLE), often simply called Llupus, is a difficult disease to diagnose and can manifest with numerous symptoms. Some of the possible misdiagnoses include depression, Bipolar Disorder, Anorexia Nervosa, Chronic Fatigue Syndrome, Fibromyalgia, Schizophrenia (a less common manifestation of Lupus with hallucinations and/or delusions), Conversion Disorder, Somatization disorder and hysteria.

Wilson's Disease (a form of copper overload) is a rare disorder that has a slow and insidious onset that can often fail to be diagnosed. Copper builds up in the liver and in the brain, usually in the late childhood, teens or twenties. Brain changes can lead to a variety of neurological and psychological type symptoms, such as speech symptoms, language difficulty and behavioural symptoms.. Possible misdiagnoses include depression, behavioural disorders, Schizophrenia, mental retardation, learning difficulty, anxiety disorders, hysteria and other psychological disorders. Physical symptoms related to liver damage such as jaundice, often appear later, leading to the delayed diagnosis.

Pancreatic Cancer is fortunately relatively rare, but this dangerous condition can be misdiagnosed as a mental condition in its early stages. Psychological symptoms similar to depression are common (including suicidal symptoms), leading to possible misdiagnoses of depression. Patients also often have difficulty sleeping leading to a misdiagnosis of insomnia (particularly with difficulty falling asleep), or some sleeping disorder, including the revere symptoms of excessive sleeping (hypersomnia). There is also a well-known list of medical conditions that are all somewhat difficult to diagnose, and all can present in a variety of different severities. Diseases in this group include Multiple Sclerosis, Lupus, Lyme Disease, Diabetes - all of these can have vague symptoms in their early presentations. Also, depression can have some symptoms similar to these conditions, and also the reverse that many of these conditions can mimic depression and be misdiagnosed as depression.

BBC News UK reported on a man who had been institutionalised and treated for mental illness because he suffered from sudden inability to speak. This was initially misdiagnosed as a "nervous breakdown" and other mental conditions. He was later diagnosed as having had a stroke, and suffering from aphasia (inability to speak), a well-known complication of stroke (or other brain conditions).

Alzheimer's Disease is often over-diagnosed. Patients tend to assume that any memory loss or forgetfulness symptom might be Alzheimer's, whereas there are many other less severe possibilities. Some level of memory decline is normal with aging, and even a slight loss of acuity may be noticed in the thirties and forties. Other conditions can also lead a person to show greater forgetfulness. For example, depression and depressive disorders can cause a person to have reduced concentration and thereby poorer memory retention.

A common scenario in elderly care is for a patient to show mental decline to dementia. Whereas this can of course occur due to various medical conditions, such as a stroke or Alzheimer's Disease. It can also be a side effect or interaction between multiple drugs that the elderly patient may be taking. There are also various other possible causes of dementia.

Although the symptoms of severe brain injury are hard to miss, it is less clear for milder injuries, or even those causing a mild concussion diagnosis. The condition is known as Mild Traumatic Brain Injury (MTBI). MTBI symptoms can be mild and can continue for days or weeks after the injury.

Although the over-diagnoses of ADHD in children is a well-known controversy, the reverse side related to adults. Some adults can remain undiagnosed, and indeed the condition has usually been overlooked throughout childhood. There are as many as eight million adults with ADHD in the USA (about one in twenty five adults in the USA). See misdiagnosis of ADHD or symptoms of ADHD.

When a person has symptoms such as vertigo or dizziness, a diagnosis of brain injury may go overlooked. This is particularly true of mild traumatic brain injury (MTBI), for which the symptoms are typically mild. The symptoms has also relate to a relatively mild brain injury (e.g. fall), that could have occurred days or even weeks ago. Vestibular dysfunction, causing vertigo-like symptoms, is a common complication of mild brain injury. See causes of dizziness, causes of vertigo, or misdiagnosis of MTBI.

Bipolar Disorder (manic-depressive disorder) often fails to be diagnosed correctly by primary care physicians. Many patients with Bipolar seek help from their doctor, rather than a psychiatrist or psychologist. See misdiagnosis of bipolar Disorder. The typical patient with an eating disorder is female. The result is that men with eating disorders often fail to be diagnosed or have a delayed diagnosis. See misdiagnosis of eating disorders or symptoms of eating disorders.

Serious bouts of depression can be undiagnosed in teenagers. The "normal" moodiness of teenagers can cause severe medical depression to be overlooked. See misdiagnosis of depression or symptoms of depression.

A condition that results from an excessive pressure of CSF within the brain is often misdiagnosed. It may be misdiagnosed as Parkinson's Disease or dementia (such as Alzheimer's Disease). The condition is called Normal Pressure Hydrocephalus (NPH) and is caused by having too much CSF, i.e. too much fluid on the brain. One study suggested that one in twenty diagnoses of dementia or Parkinson's Disease were actually NPH.

A study found that soldiers who had suffered a concussive injury in battle often were misdiagnosed on their return. A variety of symptoms can occur in Post-Concussion Syndrome and these were not being correctly attributed to their concussion injury. See introduction to concussion.

A migraine often fails to be correctly diagnosed in paediatric patients. These patients are not the typical migraine sufferers, but migraines can also occur in children. See misdiagnosis of migraine or introduction to migraine.

Patients with depression (see symptoms of depression) may also have undiagnosed anxiety disorders (see symptoms of anxiety disorders). Failure to diagnose these anxiety disorders may worsen the depression.

That we have taken a long and exhaustive look at the causes of Bipolar Disorder, those

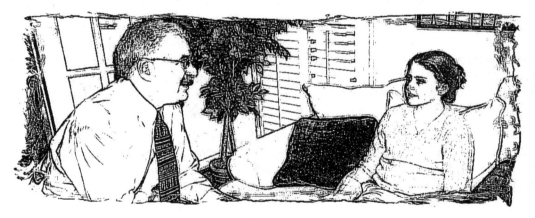

conditions that can result in a positive diagnosis, as well as an extensive list of conditions that are often mistakenly diagnosed as Bipolar Disorder that in fact an entirely different illness. Let's take a look at the next step you need to take if you feel that you may be suffering from Bipolar Disorder. You need to find a doctor that suits you to confirm, or otherwise, your diagnosis,. So which doctor is right for you? If you've realised that you have a problem, that neither you nor your support system of friends and relatives can fix, it may be time to turn to a professional for the care you need. With so many types of problems and professionals though, making a decision as to who is best to see can seem overwhelming. If you are like most people, you have probably considered visiting your family doctor (GP) for answers to your problem. While these types of professionals have a good understanding of general health issues, and can prescribe medication, they are not necessarily the best way to approach specific problems related to mental health. Choosing a healthcare provider who works specifically with mental health issues will lead to better, more effective treatment which will improve your chances for a successful long-term recovery. Learning more about the different types of mental health professionals can help you become more directed on your path toward complete emotional wellness.

Psychiatrists are medical doctors who can both prescribe medication and perform psychotherapy. They tend to look more at the biological factors contributing to such problems as depression, anxiety, substance abuse, Bipolar Disorder and eating disorders. They may look at a patient's medical and family history, and they will most likely use laboratory tests as part of their diagnosis process. If a person needs to be admitted to the hospital for tests or observation, they may also do this as well.

Clinical Psychologists are generally PhDs who are able to assess and treat mental, emotional and behavioural disorders. They handle both temporary crises arising in the face of high tress situations as well as more severe, chronic conditions including Borderline Personality Disorder and Schizophrenia. Because they are not medical doctors, clinical psychologists are not able to prescribe medication, however they are able to perform psychotherapy. Some specialise in certain types of problems while others specialise in certain demographic groups such as children, the elderly and members of the gay and lesbian community.

Counselling Psychologists are generally qualified persons who help people recognise their own strengths and resources for use in coping with their problems. They see people as individuals with differences that make up who they are. They help their patients realise how to use their gifts to their advantage in all situations including work and personal relationships. They also study how these differences affect people's psychological well-being.

Licenced Professional Counsellors, frequently found in the USA, generally have graduate degrees in counselling or psychology, although they may have more qualifications. They help people deal with issues that they have been unable to resolve on their own. Some of the issues they handle include substance abuse, stress management, grief and loss issues, suicidal feelings and family and marital problems. They address these issues, develop plans for how the patient is to deal with them and guide the patient through recovery. Once the patient is feeling more on track, counsellors also help support them through maintenance with continuing wellness plans.

Once you decide which type of mental health professional will work best in your situation, you should keep a few things in mind. Make sure whoever you see is fully qualified to provide the specific services being sought. Remember too, that finding the right professional can sometimes be a process of trial and error. Make sure the person chosen is someone that you are comfortable with and whose style meshes with your own core beliefs, values and personality. If something does not feel right, trust your feelings. Do not push for a relationship with a professional who does not seem to fit your unique needs, just because you are out of balance emotionally and do not trust you decisions. If it does not feel right, it will not work. That is not to say the process will be pleasant, but it should be comfortable.

You may feel confused and anxious about your condition. Here is a wonderful story of someone who has trodden the depths of despair, and come back to tell the story.

"I was diagnosed at 21. All through school, I knew I was different. I never quite fit in with any group. I was an outsider. I didn't know why I was so unlikeable. Then I started drinking and doing street drugs. I felt comfortable when I was drunk or high. The problem was, I couldn't handle alcohol or drugs. My behavior became so outrageous that my reputation got even worse. I was promiscuous. I had no self-respect. I hated myself. Always I wanted to be loved. I would do anything with anyone just to be loved. Love never came. I married at 19 to an abusive alcoholic. We had so much in common. Neither one of us fit in anywhere. We had a child. I had so many plans for her. She was going to change my life.

My marriage failed miserably. I tried to hold onto it. I knew I could fix it. I couldn't. I couldn't fix him. I couldn't fix myself. I didn't know I had a disease. I tried to run from myself. I followed my ex-husband from state to state trying to fix my marriage and myself. It didn't work. While I was running, disaster struck. I was having a manic episode because my ex had been out all night drinking. I wouldn't stop screaming at him - right in front of my child who was three at the time. He started beating me in front of her. I tried to lock myself in the bathroom with her, but he kicked the door in. He was hitting me in the face so hard that my blood was splattered all over the bathroom. My little girl was so upset that she threw up right in the middle of the horror.

I became depressed. I couldn't function. I couldn't feel love for my daughter. I couldn't feel love for myself. I couldn't clean house. I couldn't sleep. I couldn't eat. I was worthless. When I was admitted to the psychiatric ward at a local hospital, I had cut my wrist with a kitchen knife. My thoughts had been racing for weeks. I was convinced that my little girl was better off without me. I asked my sister-in-law to take her, and she took me to the hospital. The hospital was a nightmare. There was nobody to bring me clothing or shampoo or soap. I didn't bathe the whole time I was there. The nurses hated me. I knew they were talking about me. I smelled horrible. They all hated me. They called me a slut, and a troublemaker, and they thought I was lying.

My mind broke apart into a million pieces. I couldn't tell the difference between reality and fantasy. I had a horrific nightmare. (It took me ten years to realise it was a nightmare, and not real.) I was running around the day room ripping off my clothes. My child was there visiting with her father. I threw chairs at her and hit her and screamed at her. I made her do sexual things to me - right in the middle of the day room with everyone watching. Then I was a dragon. I was breathing fire, as I was running down the hall to my hospital room. I was knocking on all the doors, waking everyone up. I was going to buy the hospital. I was going to change things. I was going to fire all of the evil nurses and doctors. They were all frauds.

That vision stayed with me for years. I was never quite sure if my child witnessed my behaviour in the hospital. I ended up being hospitalized three times over the next ten years because I wanted to kill myself. I couldn't live with myself. I had ruined my child. Each time I was hospitalized over the next ten years, I would go into the ward, screaming that the staff had to call the police. I had to be punished. I molested my daughter! Please help me die! Once again, the orderlies and nurses and doctors were laughing at me. That woman is disgusting!

After my last visit to the hospital, I had a meeting with my counselor. I asked her to write to the hospital in Virginia where I had had my first experience at being locked up and grossly medicated. Where I had had the worst day of my life. When she received the hospital records, she told me that I had never been out of control in the day room when my daughter was there. It never happened. I could live with myself. I could live. I didn't do it.

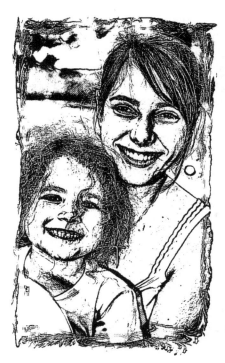

Since that day, I have been relentlessly trying to get my life back. I'm back. I am 37. My child and I lived in poverty. My ex barely helped to support our child. I was still a basket case. I felt like a guinea pig. I tried so many different medications. I had serious side effects. Over the years when I was in and out of hospitals, I went off my meds many times. I felt worse on them than off them. Finally I met a genius. He prescribed a mood stabilizer and an antidepressant. I felt better. I had another child. It didn't work out with her father, but she is beautiful.

Then Social Security Disability cancelled my income. I went to business school while working at a hardware store. I prayed. I got a job working for the state judicial department. I couldn't believe it! I was actually on the other side of the window, no longer a criminal! I had health insurance to pay for my meds and keep my children healthy! I've worked for the state for six years, the longest I've ever held down one job. I am good at what I do. I get up every morning, brush my teeth, take a shower, get my little one to school, and go to work. My older daughter is now 18. She is wonderful. She likes herself. She knows she is loved. She knows I'm here for her. She is so smart. I didn't ruin her at all. I have my own condo. It is warm and clean. I have done it on my own. I can do it.

Sixteen years ago, I hated myself. Today I love myself. I support myself. I am happy. I am not depressed. I am no longer manic. I have found the right meds. I am whole. I am writing this today because I know, from reading correspondence in your forum, that there are so many beautiful human beings out there with mental illness who don't know that there is a light at the end of the tunnel. Bipolar is forever, but it is treatable. If you are on the wrong meds, change them. If you are seeing a doctor who is not helping you, get a different doctor. Keep reaching for sanity, because it is there. I promise you. I never thought I would be where I am today. I have friends. I fit in. I am unique. I have character. I am self-sufficient. I love me. I am a miracle."

by Regina Jones

At the end of chapter 3 we would ask you to fill in a mania questionnaire, if you have not already done so. We are repeating the questioning here and you may print out as often as you wish in order to monitor your current mood and compare it with previous questionnaires to make an assessment of your progress.

1. My mind has never been sharper.

Not at all

Just a little

Somewhat

Moderately

Quite a lot

Very much

2. I need less sleep than usual.

Not at all

Just a little

Somewhat

Moderately

Quite a lot

Very much

3. I have so many plans and new ideas that it is hard for me to work.

Not at all

Just a little

Somewhat

Moderately

Quite a lot

Very much

4. I feel a pressure to talk and talk.

Not at all

Just a little

Somewhat

Moderately

Quite a lot

Very much

5. I have been particularly happy.

Not at all

Just a little

Somewhat

Moderately

Quite a lot

Very much

6. I have been more active than usual.

Not at all

Just a little

Somewhat

Moderately

Quite a lot

Very much

7. I talk so fast that people have a hard time keeping up with me.

Not at all

Just a little

Somewhat

Moderately

Quite a lot

Very much

8. I have more new ideas than I can handle.

Not at all

Just a little

Somewhat

Moderately

Quite a lot

Very much

9. I have been irritable.

Not at all

Just a little

Somewhat

Moderately

Quite a lot

Very much

10. It's easy for me to think of jokes and funny stories.

Not at all

Just a little

Somewhat

Moderately

Quite a lot

Very much

11. I have been feeling like "the life of the party".

Not at all

Just a little

Somewhat

Moderately

Quite a lot

Very much

12. I have been full of energy.

Not at all

Just a little

Somewhat

Moderately

Quite a lot

Very much

13. I have been thinking about sex.

Not at all

Just a little

Somewhat

Moderately

Quite a lot

Very much

14. I have been feeling particularly playful.

Not at all

Just a little

Somewhat

Moderately

Quite a lot

Very much

15. I have special plans for the world.

Not at all

Just a little

Somewhat

Moderately

Quite a lot

Very much

16. I have been spending too much money.

Not at all

Just a little

Somewhat

Moderately

Quite a lot

Very much

17. My attention keeps jumping from one idea to another.

Not at all

Just a little

Somewhat

Moderately

Quite a lot

Very much

18. I find it hard to slow down and stay in one place.

Not at all

Just a little

Somewhat

Moderately

Quite a lot

Very much

Remember the scoring method, the first answer scores one, the six answer scores six. The maximum possible score would be 108, generally any score above 50 should be sufficient cause for concern and you should consult a qualified medical person for a better diagnosis.

TASKS

We would also like you to fill in another mood compass, compare it with your previous efforts in the light of the knowledge and understanding you have gained about your condition.

Lastly, we would like you to write a simple paragraph, using the knowledge you have gained so far. Write down what you feel is your biggest challenge related to your disorder. Then make the best decision you are able to about what course of action you need to take, e.g. to consult the family doctor, speak to a counsellor or attend a Bipolar or Mood Counselling Group. We will be returning to this short written piece at the end of Chapter 4.

MENTAL REACTION

MIND

BODY

PHYSICAL REACTION

CHAPTER FOUR

WHAT DO DOCTOR'S SAY?

"Bipolar disorder is treated with medication, and we're gaining a lot of knowledge in this area. The fewer episodes patients have, the better the long-term prognosis is."

Melissa DelBello

Our sense of personal and physical integrity is undermined by chronic illness. The fragility and temporality of life is intimated, and the inviolability of the body and the belief in our autonomy is threatened. Bipolar Disorder (Manic Depression) is a chronic illness that displays a highly variable course and generally manifests in the second or third decade of life. Perhaps more prominently than other chronic medical illnesses, people with Bipolar are perplexed by whether they have engendered the illness and whether it is an integral part of their personality, temperament or nature. This disquieting ambiguity can be difficult to resolve and often has a profound emotional impact.

The last forty years, beginning with the discovery of the therapeutic effects of Lithium, has seen encouraging developments in the treatment of Bipolar Disorder. Although there are no cures, significant pharmacological and psychotherapeutic advances have led to the reduction of the frequency, severity and morbidity of episodes. In the following, we will summarise some of the important contemporary themes of long term treatment that we believe are important for doctors, patients and families to know.

The treatment plan for a person with Bipolar Disorder may be complex and includes consideration of several important factors:-

- assessment
- statement of treatment goals
- forging of a therapeutic alliance
- provision of psycho-education
- ongoing attention to psychosocial factors
- ongoing management of medication
- Proper assessment is an important preliminary component of the treatment and we cannot emphasise how much it helps to guide subsequent management.

For example, the treatment of a "mixed state" (i.e., an episode with an admixture of depressive and manic features) usually differs from that of a "pure" depressive episode. Initial determination of the duration and severity of episodes of mania, hypomania (a milder form of mania), depression, or mixed state is a requirement.

Further investigation should focus on -
- level of distress
- amount of dysfunction at home and in the workplace
- deterioration of interpersonal relationships
- family history
- other history of medical illnesses
- risk of dangerousness to self or others
- presence of psychosis
- need for hospitalisation (voluntary or involuntary)

Definitive diagnosis of acute states of depression and mania requires discrimination from medical causes of mania and depression (such as substance abuse or hypothyroidism) with thorough physical examinations and tests. People with a history of depression, substance abuse, psychosis or a childhood diagnosis of Attention Deficit Disorder may be at particularly high risk of developing Bipolar Disorder.

Presently, the goals of treatment are:-
- reduction in symptoms
- decreasing the frequency or preventing future episodes
- optimising overall functioning, especially during episode intervals

Treatment thus may be thought of as having three stages:-
- acute
- continuation
- maintenance

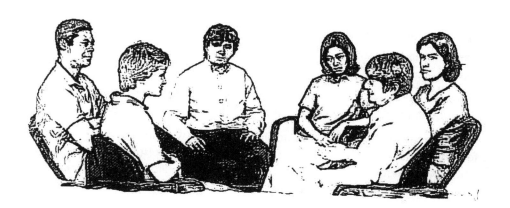

The major goal of the acute stage is to achieve a significant response to treatment. The acute treatment phase may be completed in as little as two or three weeks or it may take months to find the right combination of therapies. A complete recovery, whenever possible, is the goal of continuation treatment which may require two to six months or even longer. However, as the patient's improvement continues to consolidate towards a complete recovery, the frequency of continuation therapy visits may decrease from every other week to monthly.

Maintenance treatment, which can last for decades, is intended to prevent recurrent episodes of illness. Maintenance treatment may involve as little medical contact as twice yearly visits. The goals of this stage of treatment are best fulfilled by helping the patient to learn to monitor symptoms as potential early warning signs of a recurrent episode of illness. Teaching patients to be vigilant about their own symptoms helps to foster a collaborative therapeutic relationship. Moreover, rapid interventions triggered by such warning signs may prevent full blown recurrent episodes.

Given the long term nature of Bipolar Disorder, the therapeutic relationship between patient and doctor (or therapist or treatment team) is pivotal for establishing a solid treatment foundation.

We have found that it is best very early in treatment to address several issues:-

- course of the illness
- confidentiality
- the need to establish a contact person (family member or friend) who can provide collateral information
- frank discussion of the expectations for benefit and the limits of treatments
- the potential need for hospitalisation (voluntary and involuntary)

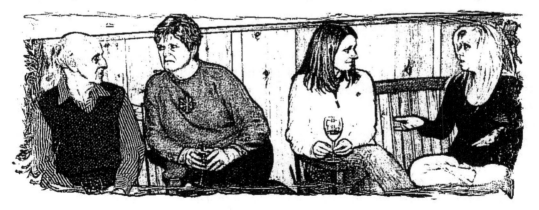

Quite often, ethical concerns emerge (e.g. poorly controlled or reckless behaviour, or the decision of involuntarily hospitalisation) and complex decisions (e.g. treatment during pregnancy or genetic counselling). As much as possible we try to anticipate them by engaging the person with Bipolar disorder and their loved ones in frank discussions.

People with Bipolar Disorder do not experience their episodes of illness in a vacuum and as a result, family, friends and colleagues invariably bear some of the disruption too. This often causes great distress. Attention to occupational, social, family and interpersonal problems together with ethical or legal difficulties is critical in maintaining long term progress. We have found that it is best to involve the family or significant others in the treatment alliance, without of course compromising the confidentiality of the doctor/ patient relationship.

The management of Bipolar Disorder almost always requires a psychiatrist, preferably one experienced with the disorder. We prefer a treatment team approach within the setting of a specialty clinic, although we recognise that such an approach may not be practical in rural or underserved areas. There are many advantages to having care provided at a Mood Disorder Clinic. There will be experienced staff who are familiar with the management and ethical issues that frequent the illness, the possibility of forming peer and family support groups and especially the provision of continuity of care.

Milder exacerbations of symptoms and full major episodes (especially mania) often unravel psychological defenses and may de-stabilise the patient or family's coping mechanisms.

It is particularly common for people with mania, despite frequent and severe episodes, to:-

- deny they have an illness
- only intermittently follow through with treatment
- resist treatment altogether

Persistent, stubborn, or intractable denial requires skilled clinicians experienced with Bipolar illness. Our impressions are that a specialty clinic is better equipped to work with people with such attitudes, helping the patient to accept the illness more easily, and reducing concerns such as suffering alone without support.

Perhaps more prominently than other chronic medical illnesses, people with Bipolar Disorder are perplexed by whether they have engendered the illness and whether it is an integral part of their personality, temperament or nature. This disquieting ambiguity can be difficult to resolve, and often has a profound emotional impact.

Medication treatment of Bipolar Disorder currently is the cornerstone of all modern therapeutic approaches, especially among long term treatments. Americans are particularly reluctant to accept pharmacologic treatments for conditions that they view as having emotional or psychological origins (recent surveys suggest that between 30% and 50% of people with Bipolar Disorder are not receiving any current medication). It is therefore not surprising that some individuals will seek unconventional treatments that emphasise macrobiotic, holistic or natural remedies. While keeping an open mind about new developments is a good general principal, we wish to strongly emphasise that the only scientifically proven treatments for Bipolar Disorder are pharmacological. We also strongly discourage the use of such natural remedies without the collaboration of a competent qualified psychiatrist.

Research and clinical experience clearly supports the use of mood stabilisers in the long term prophylaxis or prevention of new episodes of Bipolar disorder.

The three most effective mood stabilisers are:-

- Lithium
- Carbamazepine (Tegretol)
- Valproate(Depakote)

These agents are equally effective as acute phase treatments for mania. Although Lithium is usually used as the first line of treatment because of its long track record, relative safety and inexpensiveness. All three mood stabilizers are reliably measured by simple blood tests, a significant advantage for treatment. When these mood stabilisers are used for maintenance therapy they have been shown to reduce the number and severity of subsequent episodes, as well as improve mood stability between episodes.

The mood stabilisers are also somewhat effective for treatment of acute Bipolar Depression. They are generally not fast acting. They may take at least two weeks or even longer to be effective in diminishing manic symptoms and up to eight weeks to diminish depression symptoms. During acute episodes of illness, and depending on the nature of the mood instability, mood stabilisers are frequently supplemented with antipsychotic, benzodiazepines or antidepressants.

Electro Convulsive Therapy (ECT) is a rapid and powerfully effective treatment for both Bipolar mania depression. It was probably under used in the 1990's because of the stigma of Shock Treatments and because many severely ill people Bipolar Disorder depression would not consent to the treatment. The dangers of ECT have been greatly exaggerated by anti-psychiatry groups. However ECT is an expensive treatment and its major side effect, memory loss, can be transiently disabling. Also ECT only treats the current episode and does not solve the problem of relapse or cycling into recurrent episodes. Effective ECT must be followed with treatment of a mood stabiliser. Weekly or monthly sessions of maintenance ECT are recommended for people who have had multiple relapses despite use of preventative medications.

Prior to initiation of any mood stabiliser a careful medical history concentrating on cardiac, liver, renal, thyroid and the central nervous system should be undertaken.

There should be a review of present and past drug use encompassing:-

- prescription drugs
- over the counter preparations
- illegal drugs
- alcohol

- caffeine
- nicotine usage

Other areas also need to be explored for example:-

- dietary habits
- weight change
- exercise and recreational habits
- sexual habits
- pregnancy status

Additionally, laboratory investigations of medical causes of mood elevation or depression are considered. Depending on the mood stabiliser to be prescribed specific tests may be supplemented. The use of mood stabilisers during pregnancy is a complex issue and requires careful collaboration between the obstetricians and psychiatrists. In elderly patients, or those with suspected cardiovascular abnormalities, an electrocardiogram (ECG) is an important pre treatment assessment.

As noted earlier, blood level monitoring of mood stabilisers is required:-

- especially during initiation
- after any dosage changes
- after the development of significant side effects
- following clinical changes in a patient's mood

Side effects that do not improve may prompt changing dosage schedule, lowering of the dosage, or additional or substitute medications. Patient education is particularly important here.

Premature or abrupt discontinuation of an effective mood stabiliser is of particular concern and may precipitate new episodes of mania, depression or mixed states. On occasion, these new episodes may erupt almost overnight.

A small number of people are fortunate enough to have only a single significant episode of mania or episodes as infrequently as every ten years. For these individuals, a slow taper off a mood stabiliser over several months may be worth attempting after a sustained period of recovery.

But for most episodes occur in cycles of one to three years. Each new episode appears to convey added risks of suicide or development of a refractory (i.e., not responsive to medication) stage of illness. Some have speculated that repeated stressful episodes of Bipolar Disorder actually changes brain function, resulting in more severe and less treatment responsive episodes. Therefore, many specialists recommend maintenance treatment after only one episode of mania or two episodes of depression. This may be particularly important for those who first become ill at a young age, under twenty five who seem to be at an even higher level of vulnerability.

Of the three mood stabilisers, most psychiatrists have much more experience with the use of Lithium as a long term treatment of Bipolar Disorder. Lithium is a metallic element of the same family as Sodium. It is abundant on the earth's surface, and is administered as a medication frequently in the form of a salt, Lithium Carbonate. Those seeking a natural treatment cannot find a more elemental treatment in all of modern medicine!

The precise manner in which Lithium works is not completely understood. It is clear that it effects the activity of neurotransmitters, the brain's chemical messengers, and more specifically regulates the responsiveness of brain cells. We suspect that further research will reveal that Lithium works because it stabilises or helps to properly regulate brain systems governing excitement, pursuit of goals, restfulness and pleasure.

Lithium does cause a number of common side effects:-

- nausea
- diarrhoea
- increased urination
- acne
- thirstiness
- muscle weakness
- tremours
- sedation and/ or confusion

Most side effects subside or dissipate over time and dosage adjustment often helps those that do not. Weight gain, hypothyroidism and increased urination are side effects that are more common long term concerns. Longer term treatment may cause scarring of the kidneys, although this side effect does not cause kidney failure. Nevertheless most doctors monitor once or twice a year for any changes. Overdose can be a serious medical emergency and toxic doses may lead to confusion, marked morbidity and even death. However, if taken as prescribed, Lithium is quite safe. Fortunately, most side effects are manageable and the majority of people tolerate it well. More importantly, most people come to appreciate how much better they feel after taking an appropriate dosage for an extended period.

Recommended Prophylactic Treatments (also used for acute exacerbations):-

- Lithium (Eskalith, Lithobid)
- Carbamazepine (Tegretol)
- Valproate (Depakene, Depakote)

Recommended Adjuvants in Acute Exacerbations (occasionally used as long term adjuvants):-

- Anti-psychotics (Mellaril, Trilafon, Haloperidol, Clozaril, Risperdal, etc.)

- Benzodiazepines (Clonazepam, Lorazepan, Diazepam, etc.)
- Electro Convulsive Therapy
- Thyroid Hormone Anti depressants MAOIs (Parnate, Nardil) Tricyclics (Imipramine, Nortriptyline, etc.)
- SSRIs (Prozac, Paxil, Zoloft)
- Other (Effexor, Wellbutrin)

Promising future agents:-

- Calcium Channel Blockers (Verapamil)
- Moclobemide

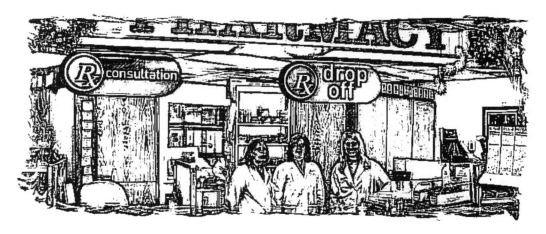

In the last decade two other medications effective for long term treatment of Bipolar Disorder have been promoted. The anti-convulsant Carbamazepine comes close to being an alternative first line therapy to Lithium. Although its usefulness to treat acute Bipolar depression is still under investigation if as effective as Lithium for the treatment of mania. Moreover, Carbamazepine is possibly more effective than Lithium for treatment of rapid mood cycling and mixed mood states. The mechanism of Carbamazepine's anti-manic action is also unknown, but it is believed to help stabilise the inner workings of nerve cells, thus modulating brain signals.

Carbamazepine and Lithium may be used together when these medications have not been effective as single drug strategies. Carbamazepine may have fewer day to day side effects than Lithium for people who have not done well on Lithium.

The principal side effects are:-

- dizziness
- drowsiness
- clumsiness

- double vision
- nausea
- vomiting

Most of these symptoms occur during the initial few days of Carbamazapine treatment and soon resolve. However Carbamazepine has less common side effects that include potentially lethal forms of anaemia, decreased white blood cell production (granulocytopenia), and a severe skin reaction know as the Stevens Johnson syndrome. Initially, blood levels of red and white blood cells are monitored closely, about every two weeks, along with Carbamazepine levels. In addition to these precautions, Carbamazepine has significant interactions with other medications and may alter their effectiveness.

Valproate has increasingly found a place as a potential alternative to Lithium and carbamazepine. Like Carbamazepine it is an anti convulsant and has been shown to be effective for mania. Less certain is its effectiveness for acute Bipolar depression and long term studies of its effect as a maintenance treatment are underway. Even less is known about its mechanism of action, but presumably it also effects brain cell responsiveness to neurotransmitters and modifies signals.

Available evidence suggests that Lithium, Carbamazepine and Valproate all have different mechanisms of action. Like Carbamazepine, Valproate may be combined with Lithium to help those with harder to treat conditions. Sometimes Carbamazepine and valproate are combined as well, although blood levels need to be monitored carefully.

Valproate's side effect profile is generally favorable and (unlike Carbamazepine) it has no catastrophic side effects in adults. (In children, however, it rarely may cause liver failure.)

The most common side effects are:-
- gastrointestinal distress
- anorexia
- nausea
- vomiting
- indigestion
- diarrhaea

Other side effects are occasional sedation, weight gain, tremours and hair loss. Most of the side effects remit over time. Like Carbamazepine, use with other medications requires monitoring.

People with a history of depression, substance abuse, psychosis, or a childhood diagnosis of attention deficit disorder may be at particularly high risk to develop Bipolar Disorder.

As mentioned earlier, antipsychotics, benzodiazepines, anti depressants, ECT and other agents are frequently used for treatment of acute episodes in combination with one or more mood stabilisers. Occasionally, for patients with refractory or unstable moods, these agents must be used for long periods of time to augment the mood stabilisers. Antipsychotics are typically used to help treat hallucinations and/ or delusions. These severe and frightening symptoms are the most disabling faced by people with Bipolar Disorder. Anti psychotics are probably the most widely used for long term mood instability. Long term usage does raise the concern of inducing Tardive dyskinesia, which is characterised by irreversible abnormal muscle movements, particularly of the face, hands and neck.

Antidepressants are used when acute Bipolar depression does not respond to a mood stabiliser or a new episode of depression develops despite maintenance treatment. The major types of anti depressants include both older tricyclics (TCA's) and monoamine oxidase inhibitors (MAOI's) and newer (selective serotonin reuptake inhibitors (SSRI's) types of drugs.

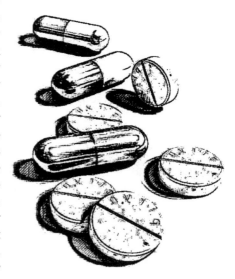

The value of the newer agents is that they tend to have fewer side effects and are much safer if they are taken in overdose. Most American psychiatrists now prefer to use the SSRIs first, although we do not think that their effectiveness has been proved for Bipolar depression. For depressed episodes characterised by fatigue, slowed thought and action, increased sleep, and/or increased weight, we still favour the older MAGI tranylcypromine (Parnate). The MAOIs require special caution however, because they alter one's capacity to metabolise a protein subunit tyramine and chemically related drugs. Thus people who take an MAGI must also follow a diet low in foods rich in tyramine (i.e., aged cheeses, overripe bananas, liver and fava beans). They must also avoid beer and most alcohol, cocaine, diet pills and certain cold remedies, Although inconvenient, most people are able to follow the MAGI diet without difficulty.

Benzodiazepines such as Diazepam (Valium), Lorazepam (Ativan) and Clonazepan (Klonopin) are given to induce sleep and to calm agitation. Benzodiazepines may be used to reduce the dosage of anti psychotics. However, they are not good maintenance medications because their benefits tend to decrease over time and they also may lead to depression. They have some potential for abuse and some people may develop physiologic dependence.

Another, often overlooked, component of long term pharmacologic treatment for Bipolar Disorder is psychotherapy. Psychotherapy may be individual, group or couples/family oriented, depending on the needs of the patient and the talents of the therapist.

Specific types of therapy include:-

- medical management
- supportive
- interpersonal
- dynamic
- cognitive behavioural
- behavioural approaches

Most approaches focus on "here and now" issues that confront people who have Bipolar Disorder.

These issues include:-

- the social and emotional consequences of current and past episodes
- apprehension about future episodes
- loss of the ideal "healthy self"
- the stigma of a psychiatric illness

It is important to keep in mind that the match of the patient and therapist may be as important as the methods or techniques:-

- does the therapist listen?
- does he/she seem to understand?
- can she/he provide a comfortable balance of structure?

A poor match with one therapist does not man that therapy per se will not be helpful.

Althoughu intuitively, one would expect that psychotherapeutic approaches would be beneficial in promoting favorable long term outcomes, research in this area is still in its infancy. Some of the areas under evaluation are the impact of family therapy, behavioural therapy and interpersonal therapy on functioning, mood exacerbations and symptoms.

Bipolar Disorder has a lifetime prevalence of at least 1%. Its severity ranges from mild, readily controllable episodes to rapidly cycling and/or psychotic states that are incapacitating. For most people, one episode of mania or two episodes of depression mean a significantly increased risk of repeated cycles of illness. Suicide, drug and alcohol abuse, and loss of family and/or occupation are not uncommon consequences. More treatment options exist today than ever before and most people with this illness can be treated effectively. For many, a long term treatment plan including daily use of a mood stabiliser, practical psychotherapy and judicious use of other medications to quell minor mood swings provides a level of benefit superior to that of people treated for high blood pressure, diabetesor other common chronic or recurrent medical illnesses.

The other major advance in treatment of Bipolar Disorder has been the advent of RCTs of psychological interventions. There is now strong evidence for the beneficial role of a number of psychotherapies, including Cognitive Behavioural and Psycho-educational approaches (targeted towards individuals, patient groups or families). Interpersonal and social rhythm therapy (which focuses on the potentially destabilising contributions of relationship difficulties and changes to regular patterns of daily activities or sleep) has also been shown to be effective in reducing the frequency of illness episodes. These treatments have been shown to be particularly effective in reducing depressive relapse.

At the end of Chapter 3 we asked you to write a short paragraph about the major problem that you felt you had to deal with, and the proposed course of action that was the most appropriate view to take. If you have not taken action please arrange to do it now, whether it be making an appointment to see your family doctor or finding out about and going along to your nearest therapy or counselling group. Once you have taken this action and have met with someone who will help you to begin the roads to recovery from Bipolar disorder, take another Mood compass and fill it in. Put the Mood compass with the previous ones and compare it with the others to try and assess the effect that taking direct and positive action has had on the way you feel about your disorder.

Next, it is time for you to understand and appreciate the enormous step you have taken by facing your disorder and actually taking action to begin dealing with it. We would like you to start a journal or diary of your moods, feelings, treatments and medication and anything else that occurs each day a relative to your disorder. Why are you doing this? Quite simply, when everything seems to be at its blackest and its absolute worst, you will be able to look in your journal and see that it happened before and you managed to overcome it, just as you will overcome it now. It is entirely possible, even likely, that after the last bad period you experienced that you recorded what happened when you came out of it. You should be able to use this to guide you to lift your emotions quicker than the last time and begin to acquire these skills and techniques to control with the very worst of your Bipolar problem. So your diary will serve both as a reminder of how you managed before, and as an encouragement to show you that you really did overcome this problem before, will overcome it again, and will learn to control your moods much more easily in the future.

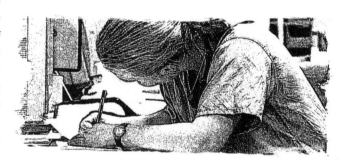

You have everything to gain and nothing to lose by keeping your journal.

- If you want to, describe your energy levels and mood status daily.
- If you don't want to write as much, you can mark down quick notes on a calendar.
- Write in your journal every day. Record your stress levels, moods, feelings of depression and medications.

- Record your sleep patterns. Write down your hours of sleep each night and feelings   of sleepiness or crankiness before you fall asleep and after you wake up. This will help you determine if your lack of sleep or sleepless nights are interfering with your emotional health.

- Write down monthly numbers. At the end of each month write down your overall moods for the month. Write down your weight and any extreme fluctuations in addition to them.

- Look at your progress. Chart your moods so that you will know when your sleepiness, abuse of alcohol or other substances and daily stress might cause your depressive moods.

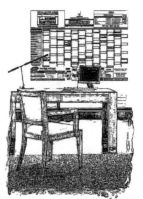

BI-POLAR JOURNAL

	ENERGY LEVEL	MOOD	TOOK MEDICATION?	SLEEP	STRESS	DIET AND EXERCISE	OVERALL FEELINGS
SUNDAY							
MONDAY							
TUESDAY							
WEDNESDAY							
THURSDAY							
FRIDAY							
SATURDAY							

CHAPTER FIVE

CONVENTIONAL PSYCHOTHERA

"We may define therapy as a search for value."

Abraham Maslow

Now that we are on the road to recovery having faced the disorder that we are suffering from, and spoken to people about it, we can move forward with further treatment. In this chapter we will be exploring both psychotherapy and group therapy, together with various options related to these therapies. We will then formulate an action plan to go forward and develop a systematic routine of treatment that suits lifestyle in terms of commitments related to work, family and financial. Also with any other considerations that need to be taken into account.

Before we go any further, you should be aware of how vital it is for you to begin some form of treatment. For someone diagnosed with Bipolar Disorder, deciding against treatment altogether could have dangerous consequences. Although treatment works better for some than for others, experts agree that it is better to be treated than not be treated. There is reason to believe that without treatment, the disorder not only gets worse but gets harder to treat. Also, statistics show that those Bipolar patients who go without treatment are twice as likely to both attempt and succeed in committing suicide.

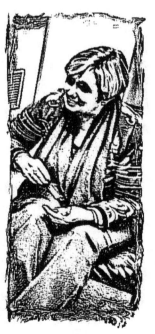

We'll be looking at the question of therapy from a medical professional. Most people have heard of the terms psychologist and psychiatrist, but not everyone is fully aware of the difference between the two. The terms psychologist and psychiatrist are often used interchangeably to describe professional people who give therapy to patients with mental and emotional problems. There are however considerable differences between the two. A psychiatrist for example will have obtained a medical degree, whereas a psychologist will tend to have a degree in psychology, often this will be a doctoral degree in psychology especially in America where this tends to be mandatory. Another important distinction is that being medically trained and qualified a psychiatrist can prescribe medication. A psychologist is not able to do this in most countries, especially the UK and the USA. There are some exceptions to this rule beginning to appear, especially in certain states in the USA, so these statements should be taken as a general rule only.

Now we know the kind of people that will be giving therapy, let us look at the types of therapy, or in this case psychotherapy. Psychotherapy is a process in which the practitioner will conduct a professional relationship with the patient to help them overcome their illness. Generally, this kind of therapy will be conducted in the practitioner's office, one-to-one and will consist of talking between the two participants. The object of this therapy is to help the patient explore the underlying reasons for their problems, in this case Bipolar Disorder, and generate and learn skills to cope with the onset of their illness. One type of psychotherapy is called Cognitive Behavioural Therapy, CBT. This has shown extremely good results and we will be looking at this important therapy in a later chapter.

As well as Cognitive Behavioural Therapy other therapies can include:-

- Behavioural Therapy
- Dialectical Behaviour Therapy
- Psychodynamic Therapy
- Interpersonal Therapy

Various other forms of therapy are being developed on a fairly regular basis. These professionally conducted therapies, as well as being on a one-to-one basis in the practitioner's office, can also be employed as family therapy where the work involves whole family or part of the family. There can also be group therapy where a number of patients, perhaps as many as fifteen, can discuss their problems in a group setting with the monitoring of the psychiatrist or psychologist concerned.

In this online age a further therapy has appeared, called online therapy. This allows the patient to have contact with their therapist, their therapy group or a combination of these using their computer and the internet. This can have many advantages, although there are disadvantages too.

Let's examine some of these:-

Advantages

- Online therapy allows people that live in remote country areas and other inaccessible places to receive therapy and information at will.
- For individuals who may be disabled or otherwise housebound, perhaps in the case of carers, it allows them to take advantage of therapy without interrupting their arrangements.
- Online therapy tends to be much cheaper than more conventional therapy and therefore is considerably more affordable.
- The anonymity that the internet offers will make some people much more comfortable with these kinds of therapy sessions.
- The online aspect of this type of therapy allows people access to a mass of information as offered on the internet.

Disadvantages

- For people with serious disorders, such as the extremes of mania or depression experienced by Bipolar sufferers, this type of therapy does not offer immediate help in a crisis situation.

- From the point of view of the therapist, they will be unable to see the facial expressions and other vocal signals and body language that they are accustomed to using as a diagnostic tool.

- Because of the non geographical nature of online therapy, there is little or no control of legal and ethical codes. Although in some cases this may not be true, where the person conducting the groups is properly qualified, in general the internet makes this kind of monitoring extremely difficult.

Perhaps the most useful kind of therapy employed in the case of Bipolar patients is group therapy, by this we mean conventional group therapy in a fixed setting, as opposed to online therapy. Group therapy is very diverse. Psychologists with different theoretical training will use group therapy for many different types of psychological problems and concerns. There are two general ways of categorising group therapy, by the time limits set on the duration of the group, and by the focus of the group and the way group members are selected.

First, group therapy can be offered on an ongoing basis or for a specific number of sessions. In an ongoing group, once the group starts it continues indefinitely, with some group members completing treatment and leaving the group. Others then join along as openings are available

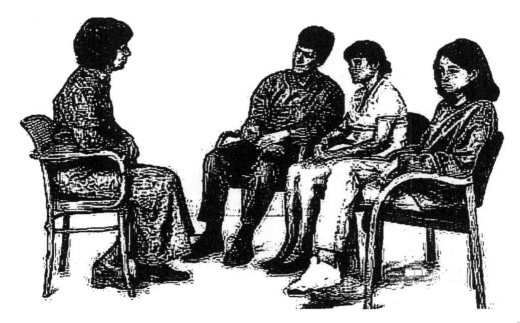

in the group. Most of these groups have between six and twelve members, plus the psychologist. There are some psychologists who have had a therapy group running for ten years or more.

Time limited groups are just as you would expect, limited in the amount of time they will run. This does not refer to the length of the group sessions, but to the number of sessions or weeks the group will run. Time limited groups have a distinct beginning, middle and end. They usually do not add additional members after the first few sessions. Most time limited groups run for a minimum of eight to ten sessions, and many will run for up to twenty sessions. The length of these groups always depends on the purpose of the group and the group membership. The psychologist running the group will structure it to run for the number of sessions necessary to accomplish the goals of the group.

The focus of the group is another way of categorising group therapy. Some groups are more general in focus, with goals related to improving overall life satisfaction and effective life functioning, especially in the area of interpersonal relationships. These groups tend to be heterogeneous. This means that the group members will have varying backgrounds, and varying psychological issues that they bring to the treatment group. The psychologist will select group members who are likely to interact in ways that will help all group members. These groups tend to be open-ended because of the nature of the group therapy process. However, some of these groups are also time-limited, but they may run longer than most time-limited groups.

Other groups are "focused" or "topical" therapy groups. The group members tend to have similar problems because the group is focused on a specific topic or problem area. For example, there are therapy groups for Bipolar Disorder, Depression, or parents of ADHD Children. Some focus therapy groups are skill development groups, with an emphasis on learning new coping skills or changing maladaptive behaviour.

Some Types of Groups:-

- Stress Management Skills

- Parenting Skills

- Assertiveness

- Anger Management Skills

Focus therapy groups can be either open-ended or time-limited groups. The skill development groups (Stress Management, etc.) tend to be time limited and usually run between eight and sixteen sessions. The single-issue focus groups (Adult Children of Alcoholics, Women's or Men's Groups, etc.) may be open-ended or they may run for a specified number of sessions.

Group therapy is different from individual therapy in a number of ways, with the most obvious difference being the number of people in the room with the psychologist. Originally group therapy was used as a cost-saving measure in institutional settings. Many people needed psychological treatment and there were too few psychologists to provide the treatment. However, in conducting research on the effectiveness of these therapy groups, psychologists discovered that the group experience benefited people in many ways that were not always addressed in individual psychotherapy. Likewise, it was also discovered that some people did not benefit from group therapy.

In group therapy you learn that you are not alone in experiencing psychological adjustment problems. You can experiment with trying to relate to people differently in a safe environment, with a psychologist present to assist as needed. Additionally, group therapy allows you to learn from the experiences of others with similar problems. It also allows you to better understand how people very different from yourself view the world and interact with people. Of course, there are many other differences between group therapy and individual psychotherapy. Many people are anxious about participating in group therapy, because they do not want other people (in addition to the psychologist) to know about their problems. Group members are told not to discuss information shared in the group with others, and usually the need for mutual confidentiality preserves the privacy of the information.

If you think about it, each of us has been raised in group environments - our families, schools, organised activities and work. These are the environments in which we grow and develop as human beings. Group psychotherapy is no different. It provides a place where you come together with others to share problems or concerns, to better understand your own situation, and to learn from and with each other.

Group therapy helps people learn about themselves and improve their interpersonal relationships. It helps people make significant changes so they feel better about the quality of their lives.

Group therapy works. Studies comparing group psychotherapy to individual therapy have shown group therapy to be as effective and sometimes even more effective. It has been widely used and has been a standard treatment option for over fifty years.

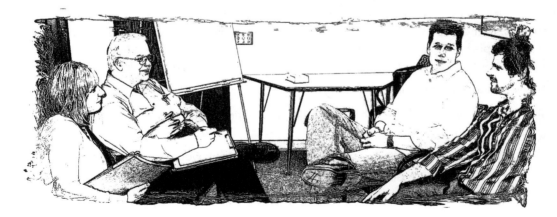

Group psychotherapists are mental health professionals trained in one of several areas:-

- psychiatry
- psychology
- social work
- psychiatric nursing
- marriage and family therapy
- pastoral counselling
- creative arts therapy
- substance abuse counselling.

In considering a therapist, ensure he or she is also qualified to lead group psychotherapy and is specially trained in this field.

The group therapy session is a collaborative effort in which a professionally trained therapist guides the discussion of the group. A typical session lasts about 75-90 minutes. Members work to express their own problems, feelings, ideas and reactions as freely and honestly as possible.

Joining a group is useful because it provides opportunities to understand one's own patterns of thought and behaviour and those of others, and to perceive how group members react to one another. In group therapy you learn that perhaps you are not as different as you think or that you're not alone. You will meet and interact with people, and the whole group learns to work on shared problems - one of the most beneficial aspects. The more you involve yourself in the group, the more you get out of it.

The time commitment depends on the type of group and the nature and extent of your problems. Short-term groups devoted to defined issues can last anywhere from six to twenty weeks. There are also more open-ended groups in which members work at their own pace and leave when their particular needs or goals have been met. Your therapist can help determine the length of time that is right for you. Typically, group therapy is about half the price of individual therapy. In the United Kingdom health care is generally available on the NHS and in the USA many people have health care insurance that will take care of some or all of these costs. In other parts of the world costs will vary considerably and you should make enquiries locally.

How do I find a good group therapist?

When talking with therapists, here are four simple questions you may want to ask:-

- What is your background?
- Given my specific situation, how do you think a group would work for me?
- What are your credentials as a group therapist?
- Do you have special training that is relevant to my problem?

Now that you have the relevant information we strongly recommend that initially you find a group therapy session. If at all possible you would be well advised to find a session that is monitored hosted by a psychiatrist or psychologist, so that you can be assured of getting the most out of the initial sessions at a time when you will not be fully conversant with how these things work and how they can best help your condition. We have supplied a group therapy diary for you to use, please fill this in after each session and keep them handy so you can refer to them as and when you need to.

Bipolar Disorder Group Therapy Diary   Week ending Saturday ....

	Sunday	Monday	Tuesday	Wednesday	Thursday	Friday	Saturday
How did I feel before the session? 1 - 10							
How did I feel after the session? 1 - 10							
How good was the session for me? 1-10							
Topic 1 that I found helpful							
Topic 2 that I found helpful							

Therapy is very helpful in treating people with Bipolar Disorder. The specific kinds of things that have been explored in this arena are substance abuse and also occupational dysfunction as well as Bipolar Disorder itself. So people with Bipolar disorder who also have problems with alcohol or substances can do very well if they actually are in a group programme that focuses on both topics. Likewise, people with Bipolar Disorder who have been unemployed, or they have trouble getting back into the workforce, can do very well if they are in group programmes that help them explore what's holding them back, and plan for getting back into the workforce.

The evidence for group therapy is not as powerful as the evidence for other kinds of individual psychotherapy, including CBT and interpersonal therapy. However, you should note that:-

> *"The treatment of Bipolar Disorder is difficult, due to the complexity and variability of the illness and the effect of the disorder on cognition, judgement and behaviour (Muller-Oerlinghausen et al, 2002). The American Psychiatric Association practice guidelines for the treatment of Bipolar Disorder recommend an integrated approach to treatment, i.e. a combination of pharmacotherapy and psychotherapy (Rothbaum & Astin, 2000); with a view to rapid and effective amelioration of acute episodes, preventing recurrences of episodes, enhancing social interpersonal and vocational functioning and decreasing the incidence of suicidal acts"*

In other words, the official view, and one which we wholeheartedly and emphatically support and endorse, is that of a multi-sided approach to the problem of Bipolar Disorder. It is very likely, even virtually certain, that no single treatment will on its own give a satisfactory mitigation of the symptoms of Bipolar Disorder. It is only through a combination of different treatment approaches that the patient is likely to be able to resolve their problems as completely as possible in order to live a happy and fulfilled life.

This story, which we hope you will find inspirational, illustrates how one severe Bipolar Disorder sufferer found help from a very unlikely source. Of course this was by no means the only source of support but to say that it helped them immeasurably would be something of an understatement.

"I was really getting to the end of my rope when by chance I made another attempt to try and learn more about my Bipolar Disorder, this time using cyberspace. I found a link for more new books about Bipolar Disorder, and by the grace of God I found a link to Electroboy.com. It happened that I was the first person to respond to the website (the book had not even been published yet). I emailed Andy Behrman and was thrilled when he emailed me a response the next day. This began a four year friendship that changed my life. First of all I loved writing and felt ready to write my autobiography by the time I was eighteen. I had such a block because I was too ashamed to write about the things that had happened to me and what I had done. I was so frustrated. Andy encouraged me and I started writing while he shared with me what he had been through. I tried to be as supportive as I could to him in anticipation of his book coming out.

When Electroboy was finally published I ran out, bought it and maniacally read it in four hours. It was that much more painful to me because by that time I already knew what a decent and wonderful person Andy Behrman was. I had faith that I could recover more fully because I saw in the book that he had done so successfully. I was grateful that I never had to suffer the horrors of psychosis and shock treatment that Andy had. I had someone that I could share psycho ward stories with, both humorous and horrifying. Most importantly, Andy was so brutally honest about his escapades and behaviors that I finally realized that this was "normal" for someone who suffers with Bipolar Disorder, and that I was not as abnormal as I thought. Now I could unlock the closet that was loaded with skeletons that had eaten me up, destroying the part of me that was trying so hard to live and love myself.

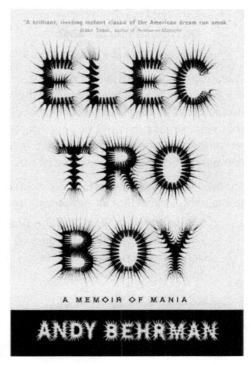

In March of 2002, I discovered on the website that his book tour was starting in Manhattan. Friends treated me to a limo for my birthday, so that after talking online for a year I could finally go and meet my kindred spirit, Andy Behrman. I am very defensive about his book, as many reviews and people that I know who have read it are "shocked" by it and judge it to be sensationalistic. The truth is, I think Electroboy makes some people uncomfortable because they can't accept their own or their loved one's illness. Many people in our society are afraid of the mentally ill in general. Most of us are not violent, and in my case I hurt myself more than anyone else. Andy Behrman has done a great service for those of use who live with this terrible affliction. I was fortunate to see him two other times over the last three years at two other book signings.

I treasure our friendship. Having a Bipolar friend who I could actually relate to has been amazing. Andy really understands first-hand what I go through, and I understand him. We accept each other unconditionally, and just the fact that Andy was able to write and publish this great work showed me that bipolar individuals can function and accomplish amazing things. I now feel that I am in the best of company; I embrace my illness rather than despise myself. I will forever be grateful for his wisdom, love and honesty in his writing and most of all for being my most compassionate true friend."

In short, you may ask:-

- Do I need a psychiatrist?
- Do I need a psychologist?

THE BIPOLAR SURVIVAL WORKBOOK

- Do I need psychotherapy?
- Do I need group therapy?
- Do I need to explore resources and options that are available online?

The answer in every case is of course yes. You need to examine every resource possible and try out everything possible until you find the treatment regime that works best for you. You will find during the following chapters of this book that we have a great number of therapeutic actions that you can take that will be very effective in mitigating at least a part of your problem. But remember the statement earlier by the American Psychiatric Association, firmly advocating a combination of therapies, a course of action that we heartily endorse.

The following was reported to us during a consultation and illustrates how alternative approaches to the mitigation of Bipolar symptoms can be useful.

"My daughter, Ann is now twenty one, but at sixteen she had her first psychotic attack. She had been very ill with bronchitis and being asthmatic the doctors had put her on steroids to keep her out of hospital. Instead she ended up in a children's psychiatric hospital for five weeks.

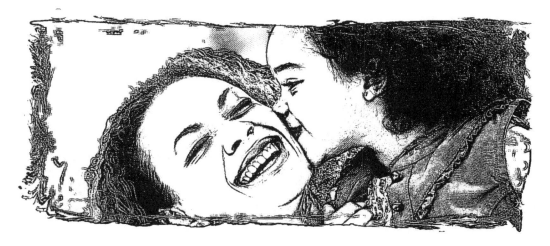

Though she never completely recovered, she went back to school and a few years later was unemployed and living on a disability benefits. She was diagnosed as being Schizophrenic. Last year her health deteriorated over a number of months and depression set in. Her psych wasn't listening to me about her many negative symptoms and within weeks she had a complete mental and physical breakdown. I had only two choices, put her in a secure mental hospital or keep her at home under lock and key. I chose to keep her at home. Love is a better healer than stress. I could not take her anywhere because she would cry and have panic attacks all the time. So we walked almost every day.

We changed psychs and medication and she made encouraging progress, but even after three months her negative thought disorder was too difficult to deal with. So one night I got on the net and looked at "Bipolar and diet". We had just celebrated Christmas and could and could tell the Christmas foods had affected her. I read for weeks and weeks about the benefits of fish oil. What did we have to lose?

Passing a health food shop I purchased the fish oil and also some Vit E (need to have them together). Within one week of taking the fish oil, her thought disorder disappeared and she is at last a happy young lady. That was four months ago, and we have not had a relapse. She is now catching public transport, doing an art course and has booked and paid for her trip to Bali with her brother and some friends.

Such a long way in such a short time!! Fish oil is beneficial to Bipolar, Schizophrenia, other mental illnesses, Rheumatoid Arthritis, hormonal problems, even some cancers, skin conditions etc. Check the net, its all there. We mix the fish oil (15ml per day) with drinking yoghurt to aid digestion and make it more palatable. Add a 500 iu capsule of vit E. We also give Ann an excellent vitamin/mineral supplement with Selenium in it. I have given out this information to many people. It is human nature to try new things, when the traditional ways dont work. I waited over five years before I found out this information (I wasn't looking for it!) I was desperate for a solution and we found it. Try it, its cheap, its good for you. Do not take if you are also on Warfarin, blood thinning medication. Find a good holistic qualified doctor. We did, he was very helpful also."

We will be looking at the whole question of diet, nutrition, herbs and other alternatives later in the book. The purpose of this is to underline how vitally important is to explore different options until you have arrived at a composite course of treatment that sees you and your circumstances.

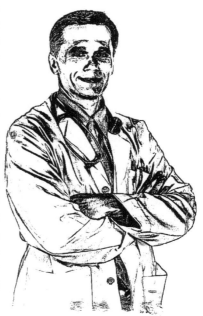

Once you have examined the range of options available, obtained appropriate professional advice and hopefully attended a professionally monitored group therapy session, you should consider a non-monitored support group. This kind of support group is called a peer support group. Peer support groups are a little like group therapy - but without the therapist. These range from ad hoc support groups formed by parents to professionally mediated support groups that may be available through a mental health clinic or public agency. Usually peer support groups do not charge participants, although a collection for snacks or meeting-room expenses might be taken up. Private clinics who run groups may carry a fee.

Biploar and other support groups use the 12-step

model or a similar self-help approach. These well known programmes bring together people with a common problem. They use methods for aiding personal change and supporting all members of the group that can be very effective. If Bipolar Disorder or indeed substance abuse or dependency, eating disorders, or compulsive behaviour disorders are additional problems for you or your Bipolar child, you may want to look into the resources available along these lines.

The support experienced and friendships made in a peer support group can be very helpful for almost any family. Peer support groups for patients themselves can also be helpful, but without adult supervision they can be dangerous for Bipolar teens. Before your child joins a support group, find out more about the programme and the other participants. Some support groups provide a wonderful healing environment where young people with bipolar disorders can share their experiences with others who have been there. In a few strictly patient-run support groups for youth, however, solid information can go missing and misinformation can be spread. That can turn support group meetings into parent-bashing sessions, or lead participants to stop taking their medications due to peer pressure.

Local support organisations are often involved in setting up, sponsoring and helping parents find peer support groups for Bipolar children.

At the end of Chapter 5 we would now like you to fill in a further Mood Compass and spend some time comparing it with the previous Mood Compass' in order to monitor your progress and the way your various physiological and emotional responses are interacting.

Do you feel you are improving, that your symptoms are being mitigated by the positive steps and actions you are taking?

If so, congratulations, move on to the next chapter with a great deal of confidence and optimism for your future progress.

If not, there is nothing whatever to be concerned with. You are taking positive steps to deal with your disorder and if you feel that it has not begun to respond to your new approach it could be that you just need to relook at the steps and information outlined in this chapter and the previous chapters. Perhaps your approach needs to be reconsidered? Or perhaps the progress that you are making is just not so obvious at this stage. In either case, once you have re-evaluated, move onto the next stage. Remember, you are taking firm and positive action. It is only a matter of time until the various threads come together and you feel the very real benefits of either a reduction of your symptoms or a complete remission of Bipolar Disorder.

CHAPTER SIX

EXERCISE

"Nutrition ... has been kicked around like a puppy that cannot take care of itself. Food faddists and crackpots have kicked it pretty cruelly ..."

Adelle Davis

Numerous studies have found aerobic exercise works as effectively as an antidepressant, helping to reduce the depressive cycle of Bipolar Disorder. In addition, exercise will certainly help to stabilise your mood and also therefore reduce the severity of the manic cycle of the Bipolar attack. Generally, the last thing you want to do when you are depressed is exercise, but even a five minute walk can help. Exercise restores regular sleep and eating, raises energy levels, generates endorphins, boosts serotonin levels and may stimulate new brain cell growth.

Studies have shown that exercise may provide an immediate mood boost for people suffering from depression. Although previous studies have suggested that exercise programmes can take weeks to improve depressive symptoms, a new study suggests that even a single workout can provide immediate benefits in lifting the mood of the seriously depressed.

"Many people with low mood, Bipolar Disorder, depression etc. attempt to self-medicate with alcohol, caffeine or tobacco to manage their daily routine. Low to moderate intensity exercise appears to be an alternate way to manage these disorders, one that doesn't come with such negative health consequences."

Researcher John Bartholomew PhD says in a news release. Bartholomew is an associate professor in the Department of Kinesiology and Health Education at The University of Texas Austin.

Researchers say most research on depression and exercise has focused on exercise as a treatment for the underlying disorder of depression. Instead this study looked at whether exercise might also provide more immediate short-term benefits by lifting peoples' mood. In the study researchers compared the effects of thirty minutes of walking on a treadmill with thirty minutes of quiet rest, in forty adults recently diagnosed with depression. None of the participants was taking antidepressants or exercising regularly.

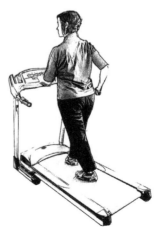

The results showed that both groups reported reductions in feelings of tension, anger, depression and fatigue. But only the exercise group reported feeling good, as measured by improved scores on "vigour" and "well-being" indicators.

The following components are essential to a safe, effective cardiovascular exercise programme. While this sets a foundation for training it is not an exclusive list. New exercisers are encouraged to have a check-up and get a doctor's approval before beginning an exercise programme.

Firstly, determine your maximum heart rate. While there are complicated treadmill tests to objectively measure maximum heart rate, most people will use a simple calculation to estimate maximum heart rate. The easiest formula is simply to subtract your age from 220. A new method, published in the Journal of the American College of Cardiology, estimates maximum heart rate with the following formula:-

208 minus 0.7 times age

Now that you know your maximum heart rate you will determine your overall training goal, and set your exercise intensity accordingly.

Determining how hard to exercise is the basis for solid training. Intensity simply refers to your heart rate during training. The appropriate exercise intensity depends upon your maximum heart rate, your current level of fitness and your goals.

TRAINING ZONES

- If you are just starting an exercise programme it is essential that you check with your doctor before beginning. After you get the go-ahead, it is recommended that you exercise between 50 – 60% of your maximum heart rate.

- if you already exercise regularly and would like to continue increasing overall fitness, or improve your times, you should exercise at 60 – 70% of maximum heart rate.

- If your goal is to improve aerobic capacity or athletic performance, you will likely be exercising in the training zone which is 75 – 85% of maximum heart rate.

While these zones are general recommendations, it is important to understand that varying your training intensity is important no matter what your fitness level. There may be times when a highly trained athlete will train in the 50 – 60% zone (for recovery or long, slow, distance training, for example). Studies show that people who exercise at too high an intensity have more injuries and are more likely to give up.

TYPE OF EXERCISE

For general conditioning choose activities that use large muscle groups and which are continuous in nature.

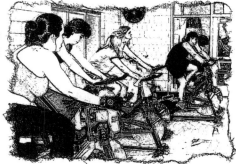

Some good examples are:-

- walking
- swimming
- running

- aerobic dance
- stair climbing machines
- ski machines
- treadmills
- cycling or exercise bikes

For those who are seeking to improve athletic performance, you will also want to use sport-specific training. The principle of specificity states that to become better at a particular exercise or skill, you must perform that exercise or skill. Therefore, a runner should train by running and a swimmer should train by swimming. There are however, some good reasons to cross train, and it is recommended for all athletes.

You should bear in mind that initially you are not looking to win a gold medal in the next Olympic Games. Your goal is to recover from problems associated with low mood and its related illnesses, including depression, Bipolar Disorder and anxiety. As we stated previously, you need to begin at the lowest possible level. Just walking up the stairs to your office is instead of using the lift could be very difficult for you if you have spent many years in a sedentary lifestyle and you are very unfit. It may be that you are suffering from the effects of obesity, which in itself presents a possible risk when you are embarking on a programme of exercise. As stated, if you plan to embark on a programme of exercise make sure that you get yourself checked out first. Getting yourself on the road to recovery from a severe mood disorder only to collapse with a heart attack would clearly be self-defeating, and could even result in premature death.

The good news is that the vast majority of people are able to find their lives massively enhanced when they begin a modest programme of exercise. People that have suffered from mood disorders find that their darkest moods begin lifting and becoming lighter. They find that their outlook on life and general enthusiasm for life steadily improves. Those people that are obese will inevitably find that there weight will begin to normalise. In fact, providing that you are otherwise fit and healthy, there is absolutely no reason why you should not embark straightaway on a limited exercise programme.

Again, assuming that everything else is equal and that you do not suffer from adverse indications, there is absolutely no downside to an exercise programme. You will feel better, look better and inevitably begin to lose some of the effects of ageing. On a simple level, somebody that lives a sedentary lifestyle is likely to be hunched and stooped in their posture with the inevitable "hangdog" expression that you will see in these people. The next time you are in a commercial area, which will certainly have a substantial population of middle-aged desk bound office workers, look for the fatter middle-aged and younger people that you come across. Look at the hunched rounded shoulders, and the expression on their faces which is generally anything that optimism and enthusiasm for the life they are leading and planned to lead in the future. In a before and after scenario you have now looked at the before. What we are intending to help you achieve is the after scenario. Upright posture, normal weight and an expression that says that this person is confident about the life they are leading and are planning for the future. It is this kind of result that we are looking to achieve by beginning to supplement your development in understanding and perceiving why you feel the way you do in certain situations. Remember the Mood Compass. The southerly point of the compass is the description of the way your body feels, which is of course is strongly influenced by your reactions both mental and physical and the resultant moods that you experience from these reactions. But at the same time your body is the whole foundation of your life.

Put in its simplest terms, the fitter and healthier you are, the happier you will feel and the more options you will have available to you as you go through life.

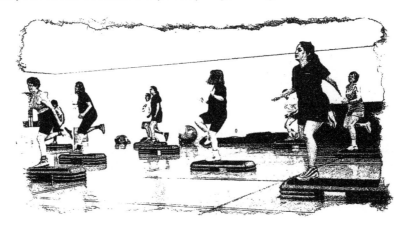

Do you need more convincing of the benefits of exercise? The average adult has two to three upper respiratory infections each year. We are exposed to bacteria all day long, but some people seem more susceptible to catching the bug. The following factors have all been associated with impaired immune function and increased risk of catching colds:-

- old age
- cigarette smoking
- stress
- poor nutrition
- fatigue and lack of sleep
- overtraining

More and more research is finding a link between moderate, regular exercise and a strong immune system. Early studies reported that recreational exercisers report fewer colds once they began running. More recent studies have shown that there are physiological changes in the immune system response to exercise.

During moderate exercise immune cells circulate through the body more quickly, and are better able to kill bacteria and viruses. After the exercise ends the immune system returns to normal within a few hours. However consistent regular exercise seems to make these changes a bit more long-lasting.

According to professor David Nieman of Appalachian State University, when moderate exercise is repeated on a near-daily basis there is a cumulative effect that leads to a long-term immune response. His research showed that those who walk at 70 to 75% of their maximum heart rate for forty minutes per day had half as many sick days due to colds or sore throats as those who don't exercise.

We hope that you are convinced enough to make at least the most moderate start to improving your fitness level by means of an exercise programme. In order to help you here is a sample exercise chart that you can use to plan your programme. It will also serve as a very valuable reminder of the progress you are making in not only recovering from a mood disorder, but becoming in the process healthier and fitter than you were before. We are also including some sample charts that had been filled in so that you get a good start in understanding what is required. Remember, whatever your preferred exercise whether it be leisurely walking in a safe local park, jogging, dancing, cycling or perhaps joining your local gym, it is virtually impossible for you not to feel better as a result and to enjoy the benefits of improved mood.

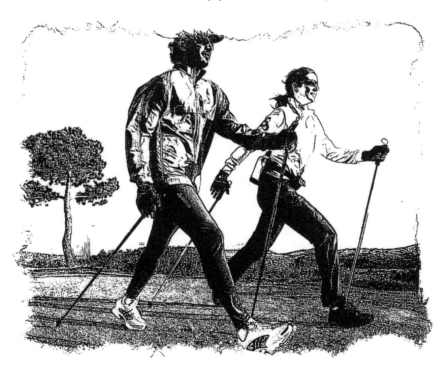

JANE

ACTIVITY	Mon.	Tues.	Wed.	Thurs.	Fri.	Sat.	Sun.
Brisk Walking	✓		✓	✓		✓	
Gardening			✓				
Mowing lawn							
Stretching Exercises							
Weight Lifting							
Jogging/ Running							
Aerobics							
Bicycling							
Stair Climbing							
Swimming							
Tennis							
Bowling							
Golf							
Other Sports							
Dancing							
Other Activities							

SUSAN

ACTIVITY	Mon.	Tues.	Wed.	Thurs.	Fri.	Sat.	Sun.
Brisk Walking							
Gardening							
Mowing lawn							
Stretching Exercises							
Weight Lifting							
Jogging/ Running							
Aerobics							
Bicycling							
Stair Climbing							
Swimming			✔			✔	
Tennis							
Bowling							
Golf							
Other Sports							
Dancing	✔						
Other Activities							

TONY

ACTIVITY	Mon.	Tues.	Wed.	Thurs.	Fri.	Sat.	Sun.
Brisk Walking							
Gardening							
Mowing lawn							
Stretching Exercises	✓						
Weight Lifting		✓		✓		✓	
Jogging/ Running	✓						
Aerobics							
Bicycling							
Stair Climbing							
Swimming							
Tennis							
Bowling							
Golf							
Other Sports							
Dancing							
Other Activities							

ACTIVITY	Mon.	Tues.	Wed.	Thurs.	Fri.	Sat.	Sun.
Brisk Walking							
Gardening							
Mowing lawn							
Stretching Exercises							
Weight Lifting							
Jogging/ Running							
Aerobics							
Bicycling							
Stair Climbing							
Swimming							
Tennis							
Bowling							
Golf							
Other Sports							
Dancing							
Other Activities							

With exercise of course goes nutrition, the other half of the equation that is the very foundation of good health and a long and happy life. There are a number of aspects of nutrition that need to be examined to be sure that your diet is optimum for you. Are you eating foods to which you have some kind of an intolerance or allergy? What kind of balance should you maintain between carbohydrates, proteins and fats? How important is fresh food in maintaining an adequate diet? Once these basic nutrition questions have been answered in such a way that best suits the type of person you are, the huge question mark is are there any foods that play an important role in helping to maintain a good balanced mood and avoid or mitigate mood disorders? We feel that there most definitely are.

Initially let us consider your basic nutritional needs. Developing healthy eating habits isn't as confusing or as restrictive as many people imagine. The first principle of a healthy diet is simply to eat a wide variety of foods. This is important because different foods make different nutritional contributions.

Secondly, fruits, vegetables, grains, and legume (foods high in complex carbohydrates, fibre, vitamins, and minerals, low in fat and free of cholesterol) should make up the bulk of the calories you consume. The rest should come from low fat dairy products, lean meat, poultry and fish.

You should also try to maintain a balance between calorie intake and calorie expenditure. That is, do not eat more food than your body can utilise. Otherwise, you will gain weight. The more active you are therefore, the more you can eat and still maintain this balance.

Following these three basic steps does not mean you have to give up your favourite foods. As long as your overall diet is balanced and rich in nutrients and fibre, there is nothing wrong with an occasional cheeseburger. Just be sure to limit how frequently you eat such foods, and try to eat small portions of them.

You can also view healthy eating as an opportunity to expand your range of choices by trying foods especially vegetables, whole grains or fruits that you don't normally eat. A healthy diet does not have to mean eating foods that are bland or unappealing.

The following basic guidelines are what you need to know to construct a healthy diet.

- Eat plenty of vitamins, minerals and phytochemicals (plant chemicals essential to good health).
- Make sure to include green, orange and yellow fruits and vegetables-such as broccoli, carrots, cantaloupe and citrus fruits. The antioxidants and other nutrients in these foods may help protect against developing certain types of cancer and other diseases. Eat five or more servings a day.
- Limit your intake of sugary foods, refined-grain products such as white bread and salty snack foods. Sugar, our number one additive, is added to a vast array of foods. Just one daily can of cola can add up to a considerable amount of sugar intake over the course of a year. Many sugary foods are also high in fat, so they are very high in calories.

ACTIVITY	Mon.	Tues.	Wed.	Thurs.	Fri.	Sat.	Sun.
Brisk Walking							
Gardening							
Mowing lawn							
Stretching Exercises							
Weight Lifting							
Jogging/ Running							
Aerobics							
Bicycling							
Stair Climbing							
Swimming							
Tennis							
Bowling							
Golf							
Other Sports							
Dancing							
Other Activities							

With exercise of course goes nutrition, the other half of the equation that is the very foundation of good health and a long and happy life. There are a number of aspects of nutrition that need to be examined to be sure that your diet is optimum for you. Are you eating foods to which you have some kind of an intolerance or allergy? What kind of balance should you maintain between carbohydrates, proteins and fats? How important is fresh food in maintaining an adequate diet? Once these basic nutrition questions have been answered in such a way that best suits the type of person you are, the huge question mark is are there any foods that play an important role in helping to maintain a good balanced mood and avoid or mitigate mood disorders? We feel that there most definitely are.

Initially let us consider your basic nutritional needs. Developing healthy eating habits isn't as confusing or as restrictive as many people imagine. The first principle of a healthy diet is simply to eat a wide variety of foods. This is important because different foods make different nutritional contributions.

Secondly, fruits, vegetables, grains, and legume (foods high in complex carbohydrates, fibre, vitamins, and minerals, low in fat and free of cholesterol) should make up the bulk of the calories you consume. The rest should come from low fat dairy products, lean meat, poultry and fish.

You should also try to maintain a balance between calorie intake and calorie expenditure. That is, do not eat more food than your body can utilise. Otherwise, you will gain weight. The more active you are therefore, the more you can eat and still maintain this balance.

Following these three basic steps does not mean you have to give up your favourite foods. As long as your overall diet is balanced and rich in nutrients and fibre, there is nothing wrong with an occasional cheeseburger. Just be sure to limit how frequently you eat such foods, and try to eat small portions of them.

You can also view healthy eating as an opportunity to expand your range of choices by trying foods especially vegetables, whole grains or fruits that you don't normally eat. A healthy diet does not have to mean eating foods that are bland or unappealing.

The following basic guidelines are what you need to know to construct a healthy diet.

- Eat plenty of vitamins, minerals and phytochemicals (plant chemicals essential to good health).
- Make sure to include green, orange and yellow fruits and vegetables-such as broccoli, carrots, cantaloupe and citrus fruits. The antioxidants and other nutrients in these foods may help protect against developing certain types of cancer and other diseases. Eat five or more servings a day.
- Limit your intake of sugary foods, refined-grain products such as white bread and salty snack foods. Sugar, our number one additive, is added to a vast array of foods. Just one daily can of cola can add up to a considerable amount of sugar intake over the course of a year. Many sugary foods are also high in fat, so they are very high in calories.

- Cut down on animal fat. It is rich in saturated fat, which boosts blood cholesterol levels and has other adverse health effects. Choose lean meats, skinless poultry and non or low-fat dairy products.

- Cut down on trans fats, supplied by hydrogenated vegetable oils used in most processed foods in the supermarket and in many fast foods.

- Eat more fish and nuts, which contain healthy unsaturated fats. Substitute olive or canola oil for butter or margarine.

- Keep portions moderate, especially of high calorie foods. In recent years serving sizes have ballooned, particularly in restaurants. Choose a starter instead of an entrée, split a dish with a friend and do not order supersized anything.

- Keep your cholesterol intake below 300 milligrams per day. Cholesterol is found only in animal products, such as meats, poultry, dairy products and egg yolks.

- Eat a variety of foods. Do not try to fill your nutrient requirements by eating the same foods day in, day out. It is possible that not every essential nutrient has been identified, and so eating a wide assortment of foods helps to ensure that you will get all the necessary nutrients. In addition, this will limit your exposure to any pesticides or toxic substances that may be present in one particular food.

- Maintain an adequate calcium intake. Calcium is essential for strong bones and teeth. Get your calcium from low-fat sources, such as skimmed milk and low-fat yogurt. If you can't get the optimal amount from foods, take supplements.

- Try to get your vitamins and minerals from foods, not from supplements. Supplements cannot substitute for a healthy diet, which supplies nutrients and other compounds besides vitamins and minerals. Foods also provide the "synergy" that many nutrients require to be efficiently used in the body.

- Maintain a desirable weight. Balance energy (calorie) intake with energy output. Exercise and other physical activity are essential.

- If you drink alcohol, do so in moderation. Excess alcohol consumption leads to a variety of health problems. Alcoholic can add many calories to your diet without supplying nutrients.

- Eat plenty of high fibre foods such as fruit, vegetables, beans and whole grains. These are the "good" carbohydrates-nutritious, filling and relatively low in calories. They should supply the twenty to thirty grams of dietary fibre you need every day. This slows the absorption of carbohydrates, so there's less effect on insulin and blood sugar, and provides other health benefits as well. Such foods also provide important vitamins.

These are simple steps that you can work towards to modify your diet and nutrition so that in combination with even the most modest exercise programme it is virtually guaranteed to lift your mood in any given situation. However, the next question we will consider, are there foods that can be helpful in lifting mood?

If you do not feel good about yourself, and do not have someone supportive to listen to, this can be a major cause of lower or altered state of mood, however good your diet might be. There are a number of nutritional imbalances that can make you prone to poor mood, anxiety and depression. These are:-

- essential fats - do you need more Omega 3?
- your homocysteine level - is it too high, corrected with B vitamins?
- serotonin levels - do they need boosting with amino acids?
- blood sugar balance - is yours within the healthy range?
- Chromium - are you getting enough?

So here are some suggestions to get you started with some of these foods, vitamins and minerals. This list is by no means definitive and you would be well advised to explore online sites to find out yourself how other people are reporting benefits from other foods of this type.

INCREASE YOUR OMEGA 3 FATS

The richest dietary source is from fish specifically carnivorous cold water fish, such as salmon, mackerel and herring. Surveys have shown that the more fish a country eats the lower is their incidence of depression. There's a type of omega 3 fat called EPA which seems to be the most potent natural anti-depressant. Again, let's examine the evidence.

There have been six double-blind placebo controlled trials to date, five of which show significant improvement. The first trial by Dr Andrew Stoll from Harvard Medical School, published in the Archives of General Psychiatry, gave forty depressed patients either omega 3 supplements versus placebo and found a highly significant improvement. The next, published in the American Journal of Psychiatry, tested the effects of giving twenty people suffering from severe depression who were already on anti-depressants but still depressed, a highly concentrated form of omega 3 fat, called ethyl-EPA versus a placebo. By the third week the depressed patients were showing major improvement in their mood, while those on placebo were not. The latest trial by Dr Sophia Frangou from the Institute of Psychiatry in London gave a concentrated form of EPA versus placebo, to twenty six depressed people with Bipolar Disorder (manic depression) and again found a significant improvement. Of those that measured the Hamilton Rating Scale, including one recent 'open' trial not involving placebos, published last year the average improvement in depression was approximately double that shown by anti-depressant drugs, without the side-effects. This may be because omega-3s help to build your brain's neuronal connections as well as the receptor sites for neurotransmitters. Therefore the more omega-3s in your blood, the more serotonin you are likely to make and the more responsive you become to its effects.

SIDE EFFECTS

In some earlier studies which gave fourteen fish oil capsules a day mild gastrointestinal discomfort, mainly loose bowels. However, nowadays you can buy more concentrated EPA rich fish oils so the amount of actual fish oil required is less. Supplementing fish oils also reduces risk for heart disease, reduces arthritic pain and may improve memory and concentration.

INCREASE YOUR INTAKE OF B VITAMINS

People with either low blood levels of the B-vitamin folic acid, or high blood levels of the protein homocysteine, (a sign that you are not getting enough B6, B12 or folic acid) are both more likely to be depressed and less likely to get a positive result from anti-depressant drugs. In a study comparing the effects of giving an SSRI with either a placebo or with folic acid, 61% of patients improved on the placebo combination but 93% improved with the addition of folic acid. But how does folic acid itself, a cheap vitamin with no known side-effects, compare to anti-depressants?

Three trials involving 247 people addressed this question. Two involving 151 people assessed the use of folic acid in addition to other treatment, and found that adding folic acid reduced HRS scores on average by a further 2.65 points. That's not as good as the results with 5-HTP but as good, if not better than antidepressants. These studies also show that more patients treated with folate experienced a reduction in their Hamilton Rating score of greater than 50% after ten weeks compared to those on anti-depressants.

Having a high level of homocysteine, a toxic protein found in the blood, doubles the odds of a woman developing depression. The ideal level is below 6, and certainly below 9. The average level is 10-11. Depression risk doubles with levels above 15. The higher your level the more likely folic acid will work for you.

Folic acid is one of seven nutrients - the others being B2, B6, B12, zinc, magnesium and TMG - that help normalise homocysteine. Deficiency in vitamin B3, B6, folic acid, zinc and magnesium have all been linked to depression. Having a low intake of these nutrients means your brain is good at 'methylating' which is the process by which the brain keeps it's chemistry in balance. So it makes sense to both eat wholefoods, fruits, vegetables, nuts and seeds, which are high in these nutrients and supplementing a multivitamin.

SIDE EFFECTS?

There are none, except lower risk for heart disease, strokes, Alzheimer's Disease and improved energy and concentration. However, if you are vegan and B12 deficient, taking folic acid on its own can mask the symptoms, but the underlying nerve damage caused by B12 deficiency anaemia can persist. So, don't take folic acid without also supplementing vitamin B12.

BOOST YOUR SEROTONIN WITH AMINO ACIDS

Serotonin is made in the body and brain from an amino acid 5-Hydroxy Tryptophan (5-HTP), which in turn is made from another amino acid called Tryptophan. Both can be found in the diet. Tryptophan is in many protein rich foods such as meat, fish, beans and eggs, while the richest source of 5-HTP is the African Griffonia bean. Just not getting enough tryptophan is likely to make you depressed.

Both have been shown to have an antidepressant effect in clinical trials, although 5HTP is more effective - 27 studies, involving 990 people to date, most of which proved effective. So how do they compare with anti-depressants? In play-off studies between 5-HTP and SSRI antidepressants, 5-HTP generally comes out slightly better. One double-blind trial headed by Dr. Poldinger at the Basel University of Psychiatry gave 34 depressed volunteers either the SSRI fluvoxamine (Luvox) or 300 mg of 5-HTP. At the end of the six weeks, both groups of patients had had a significant improvement in their depression. However, those taking 5-HTP had a slightly greater improvement, compared to those on the SSRI, in each of the four criteria assessed-depression, anxiety, insomnia, and physical symptoms-as well as the their own self-assessment, although this improvement was not statistically significant.

Anti-depressant drugs in some sensitive people can induce an overload of serotonin called Serotonin Syndrome characterised by feeling hot, high blood pressure, twitching, cramping, dizziness and disorientation. Some concern has been expressed about the possibility of increasing the odds of Serotonin Syndrome with the combination of 5-HTP and an SSRI drug. However a recent review on the safety of 5-HTP concludes that Serotonin Syndrome has not been reported in humans in association with 5-HTP, either as monotherapy (on its own) or in combination with other medications".

Exercise, sunlight and reducing your stress level also tend to promote Serotonin.

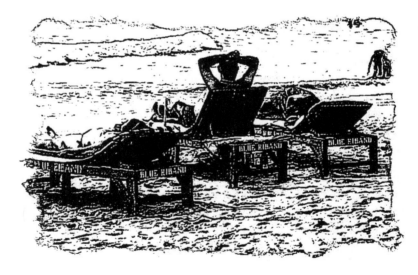

SIDE-EFFECTS

Some people experience mild gastrointestinal disturbance on 5-HTP, which usually stops within a few days. Since there are Serotonin receptors in the gut, which don't normally expect to get the real thing so easily, they can overreact if the amount is too high resulting in transient nausea.

If so, just lower the dose.

BALANCE YOUR BLOOD SUGAR

There is a direct link between mood and blood sugar balance. All carbohydrate foods are broken down into glucose and your brain runs on glucose. The more uneven your blood sugar supply the more uneven your mood.

Eating lots of sugar is going to give you sudden peaks and troughs in the amount of glucose in your blood. Symptoms include:-

- fatigue
- irritability
- dizziness
- insomnia
- excessive sweating (especially at night)
- poor concentration and forgetfulness
- excessive thirst
- depression and crying spells
- digestive disturbances
- blurred vision

Since the brain depends on an even supply of glucose it is no surprise that sugar has been implicated in aggressive behaviour, anxiety, depression and fatigue.

Lots of refined sugar and refined carbohydrates (white bread, pasta, rice and most processed foods,) is also linked with depression because these foods not only supply very little in the way of nutrients but they also use up the mood enhancing B vitamins. Sugar also diverts the supply of another nutrient we haven't mentioned yet but is also involved in mood - Chromium. This mineral is vital for keeping your blood sugar level stable because insulin, which clears glucose from the blood, can't work properly without it. (see next section)

The best way to keep your blood sugar level even is to eat what is called a low Glycaemic Load (GL) diet and avoid, as much as you can, refined sugar and refined foods. Instead eat whole foods, fruit, vegetables and regular meals. The book, the Holford Low GL Diet, explains exactly how to do this. Caffeine also has a direct effect on your blood sugar and your mood and is best kept to a minimum, as is alcohol.

SIDE EFFECTS

None

INCREASE INTAKE OF CHROMIUM

This mineral is vital for keeping your blood sugar level stable because insulin, which clears glucose from the blood, cannot work properly without it. In fact just supplying proper levels of

Chromium to certain depressed patients can make a big difference.

If you answer yes to a five or more of these questions you may be suffering from what's called "atypical" depression.

- Do you crave sweets or other carbohydrates?
- Do you tend to gain weight?
- Are you tired for no obvious reason?
- Do your arms or legs feel heavy?
- Do you tend to feel sleepy or groggy much of the time?
- Are your feelings easily hurt by the rejection of others?
- Did your depression begin before the age of thirty?

It is called atypical because in 'classic' depression people lose their appetite, don't eat enough, lose weight and can't sleep. It affects between 25 to 42% of the depressed population, and an even higher percentage among depressed women, so it is extremely common rather than 'atypical'. A chance discovery by Dr Malcolm McLeod, clinical professor of psychiatry at the University of North Carolina, suggested that people who suffer with 'atypical' depression might benefit from chromium supplementation.

In a small double-blind study McLeod gave ten patients suffering from atypical depression Chromium supplements of 600mcg a-day and five others a placebo for eight weeks. The results were dramatic. Seven out of ten taking the supplements showed a big improvement, versus none on the placebo. Their Hamilton Rating Score for depression dropped by an unheard of 83%; from 29 - major depression - to 5 - not depressed. A larger trial at Cornell University with 113 patients has confirmed the finding. After eight weeks 65% of those on Chromium had had a major improvement, compared to 33% on placebos.

SIDE EFFECTS

None, except more energy and better weight control. Chromium, if taken in the evening, can increase energy and hence interfere with sleep. Chromium has no toxicity even at amounts one hundred times this.

HERBAL SUPPLEMENTS

In general, there is not much research about herbal or natural supplements. Little is known about their effects on Bipolar Disorder. St. John's Wort (Hypericum perforatum), often marketed as a natural antidepressant, may cause a switch to mania in some people with Bipolar Disorder. St. John's Wort can also make other medications less effective, including some antidepressant and anticonvulsant medications. Scientists are also researching omega-3 fatty acids (most commonly found in fish oil) to measure their usefulness for long-term treatment of Bipolar Disorder, and report encouraging early results. (We mentioned in Chapter 5 the mother of Ann who discovered the powerful impact of fish oil on her daughter's Bipolar symptoms). It would be fair to say that so far study results have been mixed. It is important to talk with a doctor before taking any herbal or natural supplements because of the serious risk of interactions with other medications.

The research available suggests that herbal supplements can be a highly effective in the treatment of not only Bipolar Disorder but a number of other related disorders such as depression, anxiety and phobias.

In a study published in the July 2002 British Journal of Psychiatry, 172 young adult prisoners in maximum security were given supplements of vitamins and minerals roughly equating to the US recommended daily allowance (RDA), plus fatty acids. The average time for those staying in the study was 146 days. While there was no change in the placebo group, there was a 35.1% drop in antisocial behaviour for those taking supplements for at least two weeks and a 37% drop in violent offenses.

Speaking at a symposium, "Mineral/Vitamin Modification of Mental Disorders and Brain Function" at the 2003 American Psychiatric Association's annual meeting, the study's lead author, Bernard Gesch CQSW of Oxford, noted that crime has increased seven-fold in the last fifty years. Over the same period of time he reported, the trace element content in fruits and vegetables appears to have fallen significantly. According to the Centers for Disease Control, 79% of high school students eat less than five fruits or vegetables a day, and it is estimated that the ratio of omega-6 to omega-3 intake has increased six-fold since Paleolithic times.

The RDA was never meant to be regarded as optimal, more than one speaker reminded those at the same symposium. Instead, it is the minimum considered to prevent diseases such as Scurvy or Beriberi. According to a review article by Fairfield and Fletcher published in the June 19, 2002 JAMA, "most people do not consume an optimal amount of all vitamins by diet alone."

At the same session, David Benton PhD of the University of Wales, Swansea, cited his 1991 study where those who took 50 mg of Thiamin (Vitamin B1) - nearly fifty times the RDA - reported improved moods and exhibited faster reaction times, with no change in the placebo group. The study population (female undergraduates) were all well-nourished with no mood disorders.

In another study, those on 100 mcg of the trace mineral Selenium - twice the RDA - reported less depression, anxiety and tiredness.

Finally, a 1995 study on young healthy adults found that ten times the recommended doses of nine vitamins after twelve months resulted in improved performance on a range of cognitive functions in the females but not the males.

Dr. Benton related that the brain is arguably the most nutritionally sensitive organ in the body, playing a key role in controlling bodily functions. It is the most metabolically active organ, with 2% of the body's mass accounting for 20% of basal metabolic rate. With millions of chemical processes taking place, he went on to say, "If each of these is only a few % below par, it is easy to imagine some sort of cumulative effect resulting in less than optimal functioning".

Added Bonnie Kaplan, PhD of the University of Calgary: "We know that dietary minerals and vitamins are necessary in virtually every metabolic action that occurs in the mammalian brain. The brain is a chemical factory that produces serotonin, dopamine, norepinephrine and other brain chemicals twenty four hours a day. The only raw materials for their syntheses are nutrients namely amino acids, vitamins, minerals, etc. If the brain receives improper amounts of these nutrient building blocks, we can expect serious problems with our neurotransmitters."

For instance, some depression patients have a genetic pyrrole disorder which renders them grossly deficient in vitamin B6. Pyrroles bind with B6 and then with Zinc, thus depleting these nutrients. According to Dr Walsh, these individuals cannot efficiently create Serotonin since B6 is an important factor in the last step of its synthesis.

An outcome study of two hundred depressed patients treated at the Pfeiffer Center found 60% reported major improvement and 25% minor improvement. Treatment complements medications, but as the patient begins improving medication may be lowered or gradually dropped. Stopping treatment will result in relapses.

Depression can stem from any number of other conditions in the body, including:-

- hypothyroidism
- heart problems
- lack of exercise
- diabetes
- side effects of other drugs

Nutrient deficiencies include:-

- Vitamin B2
- Vitamin B6 (which can be low in those taking birth control or oestrogen)
- Vitamin B9 (folic acid).

A 2003 Finnish study of 115 depressed outpatients being treated with antidepressants found that those who responded fully to treatment had higher levels of vitamin B12 in their blood than at the beginning of treatment. The comparison was between patients with normal B12 levels and higher than normal ones rather than between deficient and normal. The study's lead author, Jukka Hintikka MD, told BBC News that one possible explanation could be that B12 is needed to manufacture certain neurotransmitters. Another theory is that vitamin B12 deficiency leads to the accumulation of the amino acid homocysteine, which has been linked to depression. A 1999 study found that both higher levels of B12 (compared to patients with deficient levels) and folate (vitamin B9 found in leafy green vegetables) corresponded with a better outcome.

A 1997 Harvard study supports earlier findings that show:-

1. a link can be made between folate deficiency and depressive symptoms, and

2.   that low folate levels can interfere with the antidepressant activity of the SSRIs.

A 2002 Oxford review of three studies involving 247 patients found that folate when added to other treatment reduced Hamilton Depression scores by 2.65 points in two studies while a third found no added benefit, leading the authors to conclude "folate may have a potential role as a supplement to other treatment for depression."

Psychology Today reports that several small studies have found that the mineral Chromium - either by itself or with antidepressants - has proved effective for treating mild to severe depression. A recent Duke University study found 600 mcg of Chromium picolinate resulted in a reduction of symptoms associated with atypical depression, including a tendency to overeat. Chromium may act on insulin, which controls blood sugar (researchers have linked depression and diabetes). The mineral is found in whole grains, mushrooms, liver and brewer's yeast.

It isn't just about mood. According to Mattson and Shea of the NIH in a 2002 study: "Dietary folate is required for normal development of the nervous system, playing important roles regulating neurogenesis and programmed cell death."

An article in Psychology Today reports that antioxidants scavenge and fight off free radicals, those rogue oxygen molecules that damage cell membranes and DNA. The brain, being the most metabolically active organ in the body, is especially susceptible to free radical damage. Free radical damage is No Iframes implicated in cognitive decline and memory loss, and may be a leading cause of Alzheimer's. Studies suggest that vitamins C and E may work synergistically to prevent Alzheimer's and to slow memory loss. The RDA for vitamin E is 22 international units (IU) and 75 to 90 mg for vitamin C, but supplements may contain up to 1,000 IU of vitamin E and more than 1,000 mg of vitamin C. In the Alzheimer's study, involving 5,000 individuals, the greatest impact occurred among those who took the two vitamins in combination. Taking either of the vitamins alone or taking multivitamins provided no protection.

Julia Ross, author of The Mood Cure, advises taking amino acids to counter some of the brain's deficiencies, including:-

- Tyrosine, a precursor of both Norepinephrine and Dopamine, can act as an energiser, and is available over the counter.
- Phenylalanine, a precursor to Tyrosine, is also an option.
- Tryptophan, the precursor to Serotonin, was removed from the US market in 1989 after a manufacturer produced a highly toxic contaminate, but is still available by prescription.

Less is more, with lower doses more effective than higher doses. Taking the amino acid with carbohydrates helps in its absorption.

Psychology Today reports that Andrew Stoll MD, the Harvard psychiatrist who put omega-3 on the map with his 1999 pilot study, is exploring the amino acid Taurine for treating Bipolar Disorder. Taurine acts as an inhibitory neurotransmitter. According to Psychology Today "The results of the study have not yet been published, but Stoll did say that it works really well for Bipolar Disorder."

Rita Elkins in her book Solving the Depression Puzzle, notes that soil depletion may account for the deficiencies of certain vitamins and minerals in our diet. In making the case for nutritional supplements, she notes:-

- Average calcium consumption in the US and Canada is two thirds of the RDA level of 800 mg.
- 59% of our calories come from nutrient-poor sources such as soft drinks, white bread and snack foods.
- The average American achieves only half the recommended levels of folic acid.
- Nine of ten diets contain only marginal amounts of vitamins A, C, B1, B2, B6, chromium, iron, copper and zinc.
- Only one person in five consumes adequate levels of vitamin B6.
- 72% of adult Americans fall short of the RDA recommendation for magnesium.
- The Journal of Clinical Nutrition reported less than 10% of those surveyed ate a balanced diet.
- Up to 80% of exercising women have iron-deficient blood.

In 1969 the Nobel scientist Linus Pauling coined the term "orthomolecular" to describe the use of naturally occurring substances, particularly nutrients, in maintaining health and treating disease. According to Dr Pauling: "Orthomolecular psychiatry is the achievement and preservation of mental health by varying the concentrations in the human body of substances that are normally present, such as the vitamins."

Orthomolecular medicine was pioneered by Abram Hoffer MD, PhD, who said in a 1998 interview, "I made a prediction in 1957 that by 1997 our practices would be accepted. I assumed it would take forty years, since in medicine it typically takes two generations before new ideas are accepted. We're more or less on schedule."

Back at the midpoint in the schedule, a 1973 American Psychiatric Association task force report used the word "deplorable" to describe the lack of hard research evidence to back the claims of proponents of high-dose vitamins and orthomolecular treatment. In light of the fact that funding for these kind of studies is virtually non-existent, however, the criticism is rather disingenuous. In fact, there is an institutional bias against studying more than one ingredient at a time, which dooms proposals for large-scale randomised control trials for multi-vitamins and minerals to death by red tape.

Thirty years later, the profession is still a long way from embracing nutritional supplements, but it has probably advanced from employing excessive rhetoric to attack its practitioners. Having said that, in today's largely unregulated market there are quacks with fantastic claims abound, along with suppliers of shoddy goods. Buyer beware is the rule.

In 2000, this writer happened to come across an item in a Canadian newspaper about an

Alberta Company, Synergy of Canada Ltd, that was test marketing a mix of thirty six supplements, called EMPower, based on a formula to calm aggressive hogs.

I ran a short item in my newsletter, McMan's Depression and Bipolar Weekly, and next thing the company was bombarded with enquiries about its product.

Founder Anthony Stephan's story is compelling, how after his Bipolar wife Deborah committed suicide in 1994, and how after exhausting all medical routes, he turned to friend David Hardy for help for two of his Bipolar children. David came up with a variation on his formula he used for calming down hogs, and Anthony administered the supplement to his kids. As he describes it:

Joseph was treated with Lithium. When he would take the Lithium he complained of severe side effects ... when he refused it, he would lapse into severe mania and panic within a couple of days.

On January 20th 1996 Joseph started using the nutritional supplementation program. He weaned off the Lithium within four days. Within two weeks, his mood and emotional control improved drastically. He has maintained total wellness, and essentially no symptoms of Bipolar since that time.

As for daughter Autumn, who first exhibited symptoms when she was twenty and became increasingly difficult to control with her rapid-cycling moods and suicidal he states:

On February 18th 1996 Autumn started the supplement program. Within four days she was forced to eliminate Haldol and Rivotril [Klonopin] because of the drastically increasing side effects. Ativan was no longer required as the mania became more manageable in the absence of hallucinations. After one week on the program, she returned home to her husband. After one month, she began the reduction and elimination of the Epival [Depakote] (used as a mood stabilizer). March 28th, 1996 marks the last day that Autumn took medication for Bipolar Affective Disorder.

Autumn has remained stable and healthy beyond her wildest dreams and the expectations of her psychiatrist, doctor and family for over four years now. In her final visit with her psychiatrist, he indicated that there was never an expectation for remission, given her diagnosis and severe and unrelenting cycles.

THE DOWNSIDE OF THE SYNERGY PROGRAMME IS THAT IT IS EXPENSIVE.

EMPower has not suffered from lack of controversy. Health Canada has attempted to shut down its operations, its nonprofit arm Truehope. Truehope works with patients and has been accused of being hostile to psychiatrists and medications. A number of patients have complained of getting worse rather than better, a quack watch group has made Synergy its great white whale, and its founders have been taken to task for making allegedly exaggerated claims.

In December 2001, however, Synergy received a significant boost to its credibility with a pilot study and accompanying commentary published in the Journal of Clinical Psychiatry. In a

University of Calgary open trial, fourteen Bipolar patients were placed on EMPower, concurrent with their medication. Thirty-three of the thirty six ingredients in the supplement are vitamins and minerals, most about ten times the RDA. After forty four weeks, depression scores dropped by 55% and mania scores by 66%. Most patients were able to lower their medication by 50%. Two were able to replace their medication with the supplement. Three dropped out after three weeks. The only side effect was nausea, which went away at a lower dose.

In her article, the study's author Dr Kaplan, noted that deficient levels of some nutrients (eg B vitamins) are related to brain and behaviour disorders as well as poor response to antidepressant medication. Less is known about trace elements, but Zinc, Magnesium, and Copper all appear to play important roles in modulating the brain's NMDA receptor (which is being targeted by at least twenty medications presently in the development pipeline). Bipolar Disorder, she speculates, may be an error of metabolism, or those with Bipolar may be vulnerable to nutrient deficiencies in the food supply.

> "There is very good work," she said in an interview, "going back to the 1950s on something called Biochemical Individuality. For example, your requirements for Zinc or B12 may be different from another person's. We are not clones. We are really very different biochemically."

In the November 2002 Journal of Child and Adolescent Psychopharmacology, Dr Kaplan reviewed earlier findings into minerals and vitamins and mood, including:

- Low intracellular calcium levels in Bipolar patients.
- Serum Zinc levels significantly lower in depressed patients, with the severity of the deficiency corresponding with the severity of the illness.
- A double-blind trail finding resulted in improved cognition.

Dr Benton's study linking Thiamin at a high dose to improved cognition and Selenium to improved mood.

A yearlong double-blind trial finding highdose multivitamins improved mood.

In an accompanying commentary to Dr Kaplan's EMPower study, Charles Popper MD of Harvard observed:

> "In view of the 50 years of experience with Lithium, the notion that minerals can treat Bipolar Disorder is unsurprising ... Depending on how this line of research develops, [we] may need to rethink the traditional bias against nutritional supplementation as a potential treatment for major psychiatric disorders."

Dr Popper notes other promising developments, including Omega-3, Calcium, Chromium, Inositol, amino acids, and high-dose multi-vitamins.

Dr Popper in his commentary mentioned using the supplement to treat tewenty two Bipolar patients, nineteen who showed a positive response, eleven who have been stable for nine

months without drugs.

Dr Popper, who co-chaired the APA symposium mentioned at the beginning of this article, observed that while nutrient supplements are probably safer than psychiatric drugs, one should be mindful of toxic levels and special circumstances. For example, high doses of vitamin A need to be avoided in pregnant women owing to risk of fetal harm.

The issue of interactions with meds was raised, but Dr Kaplan expressed her dissatisfaction with the term, interaction. Her theory is that nutritional supplements may improve the performance of metabolic pathways, thus amplifying the positive and negative effects of medication. As a result, therapeutic doses of medication can become overdoses. Truehope advises that new users will experience initial side effects from their medication thanks to the amplification factor, and urges patients to work with their doctor in lowering their medication doses. Overenthusiastic Truehope people may say you need to eventually go off all your medication, but just two patients in Dr Kaplan's small study and only half of Dr Popper's patients achieved this result.

If you are considering therapy with vitamins or other nutrients, do so with your psychiatrist being aware of this. Since "integrative psychiatrists" are a rarity, it is wise to seek nutritional expertise from another source. It also pays to ensure that your psychiatrist is open-minded about nutritional supplements and would consider adjusting your medication if you responded well to your new regimen. Keep in mind that the final decision regarding lowering medication is one to be made between you and your psychiatrist, not with the person who is advising you on nutrition.

You do need to be careful when introducing herbal supplements into your diet for therapeutic reasons. Apart from interactions between themselves and with possible medication is that you may be taking, if you introduce a herbal supplement on an ad hoc basis it will be difficult, if not impossible, for you to monitor whether they are effective or otherwise. For this reason we have produced a chart for you to utilise in order to monitor the herbs that you take and keep a record of exactly what you have taken, when you took it and how you felt following the taking of this herb.

TASK

At the end of Chapter 6 your task is firstly to print out our exercise and nutrition charts of the examples through this chapter and begin planning your own programme of improved nutrition and exercise. You must take it slowly, at least to begin with. If you try to rush into a heavy exercise programme the end result will either be the opposite of what you are trying to achieve. You could find that your mood is lowered rather than the opposite because of the excessive demands you put on your body. In a similar way with a diet, and possibly supplement programme, a sudden change could upset your system and metabolism so again it has the opposite effect from what you are seeking. You may experience a lowered mood rather than an increased feeling of well-being. A slow and gentle approach will give your body and mind time to adjust and really reap the benefits of the positive changes you are making to it.

Once you have completed the work on your exercise and nutrition charts, you should then start looking at the whole question of herbal supplements. In any event, this may well be a long process, a process of trying out the most likely herbal supplements one by one and monitoring their effect in your treatment programme. Do this with your therapist and keep a record chart and you will be able to assess the quickest and most effective herbal therapy that suits you. There is no need to rush into your herbal supplement programme, just keep it going as a background part of your therapy. It is likely to take many months before you fully eliminate the unhelpful herbs and identify the ones that are most useful to you. At the same time you may be lucky, it could be that one of the first herbal supplements that you try is of considerable help to you just as the fish oil was for Ann.

Please fill in a further Mood Compass, and keep it with the others.

MIND

PHYSICAL   MENTAL
REACTION   REACTION

BODY

Day	Date	Weight (lbs)
0		
1		
2		
3		
4		
5		
6		
7		
8		
9		
10		
11		
12		
13		
14		
15		
16		
17		
18		
19		
20		

Day	Date	Weight (lbs)
21		
22		
23		
24		
25		
26		
27		
28		
29		
30		
31		
32		
33		
34		
35		
36		
37		
38		
39		
40		
41		

Day	Date	Weight (lbs)
42		
43		
44		
45		
46		
47		
48		
49		
50		
51		
52		
53		
54		
55		
56		
57		
58		
59		
60		
61		
62		

Nutrition Journal	Sunday	Monday	Tuesday	Wednesday	Thursday	Friday	Saturday
Meal One	Cals · Fat Grams · Time	Cals · Fat Grams · Time	Cals · Fat Grams · Time	Cals · Fat Grams · Time	Cals · Fat Grams · Time	Cals · Fat Grams · Time	Cals · Fat Grams · Time
Meal Two	Cals · Fat Grams · Time	Cals · Fat Grams · Time	Cals · Fat Grams · Time	Cals · Fat Grams · Time	Cals · Fat Grams · Time	Cals · Fat Grams · Time	Cals · Fat Grams · Time
Meal Three	Cals · Fat Grams · Time	Cals · Fat Grams · Time	Cals · Fat Grams · Time	Cals · Fat Grams · Time	Cals · Fat Grams · Time	Cals · Fat Grams · Time	Cals · Fat Grams · Time
Meal Four	Cals · Fat Grams · Time	Cals · Fat Grams · Time	Cals · Fat Grams · Time	Cals · Fat Grams · Time	Cals · Fat Grams · Time	Cals · Fat Grams · Time	Cals · Fat Grams · Time
Meal Five	Cals · Fat Grams · Time	Cals · Fat Grams · Time	Cals · Fat Grams · Time	Cals · Fat Grams · Time	Cals · Fat Grams · Time	Cals · Fat Grams · Time	Cals · Fat Grams · Time
Total	Cals · Fat Grams · Time	Cals · Fat Grams · Time	Cals · Fat Grams · Time	Cals · Fat Grams · Time	Cals · Fat Grams · Time	Cals · Fat Grams · Time	Cals · Fat Grams · Time

HERBAL SUPPLEMENT CHART

(example) HERB /SUPP NAME	Sunday Effective? 1 - 10	Monday Effective? 1 - 10	Tuesday Effective? 1 - 10	Wednesday Effective? 1 - 10	Thursday Effective? 1 - 10	Friday Effective? 1 - 10	Saturday Effective? 1 - 10
Fish Oil							
Vit B6							
St Johns Wort							
Gingko Biloba							

CHAPTER SEVEN

REDUCE STRESS, REDUCE BIPOLAR DISORDER

"The life of inner peace, being harmonious and without stress, is the easiest type of existence."

Norman Vincent Peale

Managing your stress is extremely important as stress can easily trigger an episode of Bipolar Disorder, either manic or depressive. There is a great range of stress reduction techniques.

They could include:-

- exercise
- meditation
- deep breathing
- guided imagery
- soft music

Firstly, remove yourself from all stressful situations when possible. The most common response to this stress is to ignore it and carry on regardless. However, it is highly unlikely that ignoring the problem will just make it go away. It is very likely that ignoring the problem of stress will just add that to build up further and further until the point where the onset of Bipolar symptoms becomes very severe indeed.

As a general rule, stress is a physical phenomenon that causes bodily or mental unrest.

It can be caused by big changes in one's life, such as:-

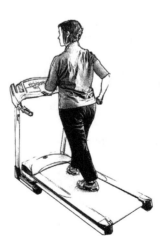

- marriage
- pregnancy
- wedding
- relocation to a new school
- death of a loved one

Workplace pressures, such as work overload, conflicts with colleagues or boss, or competition can also give rise to a lot of stress. Certain environmental factors, including financial problems, parenting, family issues, travel or other disappointments may also lead to stress.

Such stress can give rise to a number of symptoms, including:-

- anxiousness
- irritability
- forgetfulness
- low self-esteem
- nervousness
- impulsive actions

One of the most vital paths to manage stress is through maintaining robust social support systems. Spouses, children, parents, friends, business associates, associates and neighbours are all part of our social system. Particularly, prioritising tasks and avoiding over commitment are urgent measures that make sure that one is not overscheduled. You can employ a calendar or planner to plan and commit any task. You can also keep a diary and note where you waste time. Moreover, you need to plan much ahead to avoid procrastination.

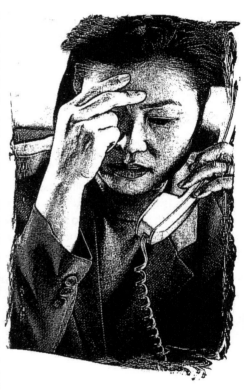

Meditation and relaxation strategies help control stress and improve psychological and physical well being. It is feasible to learn these methods in a class or at home. Audio and video CDs of these techniques are readily available. Eat healthily, see sections in this book that cover the areas of diet and nutrition. Also, you should have a good sleep daily. Develop hobbies such as gardening, photography, scrapbooking, drawing painting, writing or playing games. These are effective ways to reduce stress. Have a positive angle and be optimistic. Overcoming perfectionism and have a feeling of humour. All of them will help you overcome stress.

Avoid getting into bad habits such as excessive alcoholic intake, betting or substance abuse. Such habits only complicate matters further and increase private conflicts. The last thing you need in your life is conflict or complications

Indeed mitigating the symptoms of Bipolar Disorder involve removing conflict and complication, rather than adding to it. In case of persistent stress symptoms, you may see a consultant. The consultant will access the effects of stress on the physical functioning and stress in order to combat such negative influences.

One can also consider stress-management support from a therapist. A counsellor would identify the areas in your life that lead to stress and then work on strategies to manipulate your most stressed scenarios or moments. Thus, you can easily manage levels of these simple stress management tips. You need not do any of them especially. Just make them your habit and they would come to your naturally after that. These simple lifestyle changes would surely help you lead a stress free life.

From a technical standpoint, there has been an extremely important milestone study that links stress, chemicals in the brain and the symptoms of Bipolar Disorder. Here is an excerpt from the study.

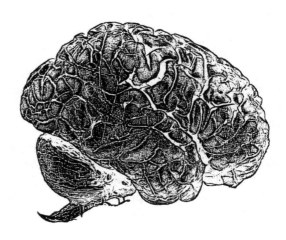

An errant enzyme linked to Bipolar Disorder, in the brain's prefrontal cortex, impairs cognition under stress, an animal study shows. The disturbed thinking, impaired judgment, impulsivity, and distractibility seen in mania, a destructive phase of Bipolar Disorder, may be traceable to overactivity of protein kinase C (PKC), suggests the study, funded by the National Institutes of Health's (NIH) National Institute of Mental Health (NIMH) and National Institute on Aging (NIA), and the Stanley Foundation. It explains how even mild stress can worsen cognitive symptoms, as occurs in Bipolar Disorder, which affects two million Americans.

Abnormalities in the cascade of events that trigger PKC have also been implicated in Schizophrenia. Amy Arnsten, Ph.D. and Shari Birnbaum, Ph.D. of Yale University, and Husseini Manji, M.D., of NIMH, and colleagues, report on their discovery in the October 29, 2004 issue of Science.

> "Either direct or indirect activation of PKC dramatically impaired the cognitive functions of the prefrontal cortex, a higher brain region that allows us to appropriately guide our behavior, thoughts and emotions," explained Arnsten. "PKC activation led to a reduction in memory-related cell firing, the code cells use to hold information in mind from moment-to-moment. Exposure to mild stress activated PKC and resulted in prefrontal dysfunction, while inhibiting PKC protected cognitive function."
>
> "In the future, drugs that inhibit PKC could become the preferred emergency room treatments for mania," added Manji, currently Director of NIMH's Mood and Anxiety

Disorders Program, who heads a search for a fast-acting anti-manic agent. "All current treatments — Lithium, Valproate, Carbamazepine and antipsychotics — take days, if not weeks, to work. That's because they're likely acting far upstream of where a key problem is, namely in the PKC pathway. Since PKC inhibitors could act more directly, they might quench symptoms more quickly. Patients could carry PKC inhibitors and take them preventively, as soon as they sense a manic episode coming on."

Clinical trials of a PKC inhibitor, the anti-cancer drug Tamoxifen, are currently underway in Bipolar Disorder patients. However, these may be more important for proof-of-concept than therapeutic utility, according to Manji, who says side effects will likely rule out Tamoxifen itself as a practical treatment for mania. "While there are likely other pathways involved, PKC appears to be very important for bipolar disorder," he noted.

The fact that the current anti-manic drugs ultimately reduce PKC activity suggests that PKC may be a final common target of these treatments and may play a key role in Bipolar Disorder. Studies have also found signs of increased PKC activity in Bipolar patients' blood platelets and in the brain cells of deceased patients. Susceptibility to Bipolar Disorder may involve variants of genes that code for a key PKC precursor and for a stress-sensitive signaling protein that normally puts the brakes on PKC activity.

The new study shows how PKC triggers cognitive symptoms in response to stress. When the stress-sensitive messenger chemical norepinephrine binds to receptors on cell membranes in the prefrontal cortex, it activates PKC through a cascade of events. The enzyme then travels out to the cell membrane, opening ion channels that heighten the cell's excitability, and stoking protein machinery that propels neurotransmitters into the synapse. PKC also moves into the cell's nucleus, where it turns-on genes.

To tease out PKCs role, the researchers selectively targeted the prefrontal cortex in rats and monkeys performing working memory tasks with PKC activators, inhibitors, norepinephrine-like and stress inducing drugs — alone and in combination. They also found that by blocking PKC, the anti-manic drugs Lithium and Carbamazepine protected monkeys' prefrontal cortex functioning from impairment by a norepinephrnine-like drug. The researchers traced impairment to a reduction in memory-related firing of single cells in the prefrontal cortex, which was reversible by a PKC inhibitor.

Genetic and biochemical studies indicate that PKC may also be overactive in the brains of patients with Schizophrenia. Antipsychotics, which are used to treat Bipolar Disorder as well as Schizophrenia, block receptors in the brain that activate PKC.

What does this mean for you? Quite simply, that Bipolar sufferers, as well as patients suffering from other disorders, should be aware of the potential damage that stress can do clinically to their symptoms. So read on and make certain that you develop the soundest possible strategies for dealing with your stress. In any case, quite apart from the reduction in the severity of Bipolar symptoms, a stress free life is a happier, more relaxed and much more fulfilled life.

Cut the stress, cut the illness and go out and enjoy yourself!

A - Z FOR REDUCING STRESS

A is for Anxiety

Anxiety is a strong feeling of unease, a state of being troubled. It can be an intense feeling of apprehension or fear about events or situations that a sufferer is facing, for example job loss, relationship breakdown, meeting new people, or life changes. Such feelings make it difficult to cope with life and are accompanied by physical symptoms too such as butterflies in your tummy, trembling hands, heavy sweating, racing pulse and palpitations. Tiredness is also a problem because sufferers find it very difficult to sleep. Anxiety certainly is not incurable and there are steps you can take to combat anxiety without taking powerful drugs. Understanding your anxiety – especially what causes anxiety – is important and there are also many skills you can acquire that will help you to cope with all of life's trials and tribulations so anxiety is not triggered.

B is for Bipolar Disorder

Bipolar Disorder was commonly referred to as "Manic Depression". Bipolar Disorder is the fluctuation between extreme moods. So, a sufferer will feel periods of overwhelming joy and elation, where confidence is very high, energy levels are high and they're constantly "on the go", moving from one thing to another. Because of the intensity of the high, judgement is impaired and decisions can be made that have serious consequences, such as a change of job, a house move or relationship choices. The second phase of Bipolar is the depressive phase where sufferers have little self confidence, low energy levels and experience little pleasure in anything life has to offer. Feelings of helplessness and despair also occur and exhaustion will also be present as these strong emotions make it difficult to sleep. As with anxiety, there are many natural steps you can take that help enormously with Bipolar Disorder so sufferers can cope better without taking antidepressants.

C is for Chronic

Many people who suffer from stress, depression and anxiety often describe their condition as chronic. However, the majority of sufferers use the word chronic incorrectly. If you suffer from chronic stress, chronic depression or chronic anxiety, it does not mean that you are experiencing severe stress, severe depression or severe anxiety. It means that stress, depression or anxiety are ongoing for a prolonged amount of time. Being under major stress at work for a month is not chronic stress, most people will experience such stress and as soon as the situation is resolved, the stress goes away. But being under major stress month in month out is chronic stress. The word chronic does not describe the intensisty, it's more about the length of time a sufferer experiences these problems.

D is for Depression

Depression is a growing problem with one in twenty people suffering a depressive episode at one

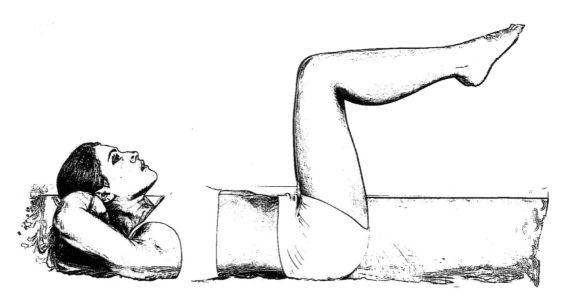

or more stages of their lives. Depression is more than just the blues. It is a number of emotions and feelings that take a sufferer to a sad, lonely and desperate place. Levels of confidence and self esteem plummet, giving rise to feelings of helplessness, loneliness, extreme exhaustion and fear of the future. Sufferers can find even the smallest of daily tasks too difficult and in this state, finding an answer to even the smallest of problems is very hard. Concentration levels are affected badly and gradually, a sufferer will retreat to their own world, isolating themselves from loved ones and society, further exacerbating the depression. Even if depression is severe, there are lots of things you can do for depression, particularly cognitive therapy, natural remedies and effective life skills to help a sufferer cope effectively with the circumstances they face in life. Gaining control is a key skill, and will help a sufferer enormously.

E is for Exercise

Exercise brings enormous benefits to our physical health. Exercise builds and maintains strong muscles, burns off excess calories, tones the whole body and gives us a buzz due to the release of feel good endorphins into the system. It can also help to maintain mental health, but exercise is not a cure for stress, anxiety and depression. Exercise does not treat the root cause and if a sufferer does exercise, it will only provide temporary relief.

F is for Food

Surf the internet looking for the root cause of stress, depression and anxiety and you will find many sites claiming that a nutritionally deficient diet is the main reason for mental health problems. In particular, they will claim that too much junk food in the diet is the real culprit. This is a fallacy, plain and simple. The food you eat – whether you eat a very healthy diet low

in fat and high in fresh fruit and vegetables or a junk food diet full of pizzas, burgers, fries and ice cream – will not cause stress, depression or anxiety nor will food cure stress, depression or anxiety. This is simply demonstrated by asking: Does everybody who eats a poor diet suffer from stress, depression or anxiety? We can also ask: Does everybody who eats a very healthy diet enjoy immunity from stress, depression and anxiety? The answer is the same for both: NO! A healthy diet is important for good health, but it doesn't help much with stress, depression and anxiety.

G is for Guilt

Without doubt, guilt is one of the most self-destructive of human emotions. Guilt simply has no other purpose other than to make the individual seriously unhappy. Guilt is a big part of stress, anxiety and depression and learning how to deal with it is important. Guilt arises out of a feeling of remorse or regret for something you either did or did not do. It is a no-win deal if you indulge it because you are always damned if you do or damned if you don't. No matter what you do, guilt will always beat you up about it. When you eliminate guilt from your life, you'll feel like a millstone has been lifted from around your neck.

H is for Happiness

Happiness is something everyone has the right to experience. It is arguably what we all strive to attain in life. The feeling that we have a good life, are making a contribution, have people to love and people who love us is a very important feeling for a human being to have. Unfortunately, happiness has many enemies – stress, anxiety and depression especially. These problems bring doubt, insecurity, fear, guilt, negativity, helplessness and uncertainty into our lives and these feelings make it very hard for you to enjoy happiness. What is very important to know is that all of these enemies of happiness can be dealt with and when you do, your levels of happiness will increase dramatically.

I is for Imagination

Your imagination is one of the most powerful things you possess as a human being. Imagination can spur you on to achieve great things. Imagination has been behind all of the great achievements of humanity. The great cities, the great discoveries and inventions, the advances in medical care, and the conquest of space all came from the visions of imaginative human beings. But imagination can also make your life a living hell by conjuring up all kinds of nasty and unpleasant scenarios that only reside in one place, your mind. So powerful can your imagination be that these highly emotive, frightening and catastrophic outcomes can be enough to cause descent into mental breakdown, even though these imaginings have not and will not occur in reality. That is precisely what happens to millions of people who let their imagination run wild and unchecked. Another important skill in dealing with stress, depression and anxiety is to make your imagination work for you and not against you.

J is for Journal

One of the most helpful things you can do to find relief from stress, anxiety and depression is

133

to keep a journal. In it you can write your thoughts, ideas, dreams, ambitions, diet and possible triggers. But a word of caution, do not continually write about things and events from your past. Dwelling on the past can be a real problem, especially for depression sufferers, so make your journal a record of more positive aspects. Keep it solely for your eyes only. Your journal is about you for you, so keep it in a place where prying eyes will not find it.

K is for Knowledge

Perhaps the most important step you can take towards relieving stress, anxiety and depression permanently is to acquire as much knowledge as you can about all of these harrowing problems. It has been demonstrated over and over again that people who understand the causes come out of their torment quickly and permanently. Of course, acquiring the knowledge is one thing, applying it is another. Knowledge is not power, applied knowledge is and once you know exactly what is happening to you, you can then acquire the skills that will bring relief from stress, depression and anxiety once and for all.

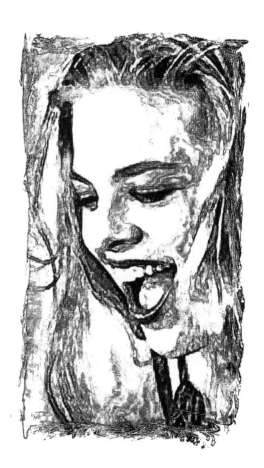

L is for Laughter

Laughter is a fantastic stress buster and is also beneficial to our overall well-being as it releases feel good hormones into our system. Try not to take life too seriously and maintain a sense of humour, no matter how trying life becomes. A great stress relief tip is to have a comedy night once or twice or month. Get in your favourite nibbles, open a beer or a good bottle of wine and watch DVDs of your favourite comedies. Just forget the world for a night and enjoy a good laugh!

M is for Makeover

A makeover is one of the best ways to give your mental health a boost, especially if you have just experienced a major change in your life such as a relationship breakdown or a loss of a job. You can have a change of style, your hair, your clothes, start a fitness routine, start a new course or move somewhere new and start afresh. You could give your home a makeover. Perhaps a new colour scheme, new furniture or clear out all of your old junk. It is effective because it draws a line under the past and you wipe the slate clean and start afresh. A makeover is a great way to deal with stress, anxiety and depression. There is something so exciting about re-inventing yourself and you can do it as often as you want.

N is for Nervous Breakdown

A nervous breakdown occurs when you can no longer cope with the circumstances you are faced with. Nervous breakdown was the term used in the past to describe anxiety, depression and stress. When you breakdown you simply cannot function, you are totally overwhelmed and cannot take anymore. This is how stress, anxiety and depression affect you if they go unchecked. If you are at this point you can get your life back. There are answers, solutions and options and there are many, many things you can do to bounce back from a nervous breakdown.

O is for Optimism

Mental health problems such as anxiety, depression and stress are not untreatable. There are a number of techniques, methods and skills that help enormously and you do not have to take antidepressants or other medications. So, no matter how far into stress, anxiety or depression you are, you have optimism. You are not helpless and the situation is not hopeless because you can and will overcome these problems.

P is for Psychosis

Psychosis is where a sufferer has thinking processes that are wholly out of step with reality. They will be deluded about their abilities and circumstances and may also experience visions and hallucinations. Psychosis is more a part of severe mental illnesses, such as Schizophrenia. It is not a part of stress, depression or anxiety.

Q is for Questions

Questions are one of the most effective ways to relieve stress, anxiety and depression. One of the most common symptoms of stress, depression and anxiety is to assign single, worst-outcome or even catastrophic meanings to the events and circumstances you are confronted with in your life. Once these meanings are assigned, sufferers will take them as absolute truths and in doing so, they trigger powerful feelings within themselves that increase the torment. So, every time you assign a meaning to an event, question it.

The following three questions will help:-
- Is this a true reflection of what is happening?
- Are there other possible outcomes?
- How I can I create more possible outcomes?

It is so important to ask questions about the meanings you assign to events. Doing so will relieve

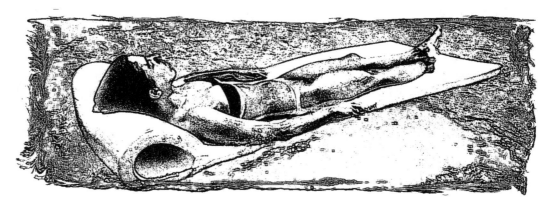

stress, anxiety and depression by lessening the impact of single, negative meanings.

R is for Relaxation

You may be aware of the saying "All work and no play makes Jack a dull boy". It is so true and in today's busy world, many people are working far too hard. Long hours, heavy workload and a lack of rest is a recipe for stress, depression and anxiety.

S is for Stress

Stress is the feeling of being under great strain, high tension or intense pressure. When you are stressed, you can find it difficult to cope. Everyday problems become difficult to solve and you can also feel overwhelmed by an event or events. Feelings of helplessness and hopelessness can creep in and there is also a fear of a bad outcome to events. You can see how such symptoms can place a sufferer under severe emotional turbulence and how these symptoms can soon descend into episodes of anxiety and depression. Left untreated, stress, depression and anxiety can be lethal and these illnesses are predicted as being the number one killers of the 21st century. Learning how to deal effectively with stress, depression and anxiety is one of the most important skills anyone can possess.

T is for Talking

When you are suffering the torment of stress, depression and anxiety, the urge to shut out society and retreat into your own solitary world can be overwhelming. Isolation further exacerbates the suffering. It is so important to keep at least one person close to you who you can confide in and talk about how you feel. There is no need to be with them every day or every night, but do have someone close to you who you can talk to in confidence. Keeping your feelings and troubles inside you just builds up pressure and deepens your suffering. Have one special person who you can confide in and they will help you get through this.

U is for Unnatural

There are numerous so-called cures for depression, stress and anxiety that are unnatural. In the vast majority of cases they are nothing more than snake-oil. Herbs, supplements, vitamins, incense – none of these will cure you. The may offer comfort, but a cure is beyond them because they do not address the root cause. Drug therapy also fails because of this problem. Drugs address a theory of chemical imbalances in the brain, despite no clear evidence to support this theory. The only way to find permanent relief from stress, depression and anxiety is to treat the root cause and that lies in the way you make sense out of every event you are confronted with in your life. This can be treated naturally, without drugs, ECT, potions and supplements and once you know how - stress, depression and anxiety will never spoil your life ever again.

V is for Vocabulary

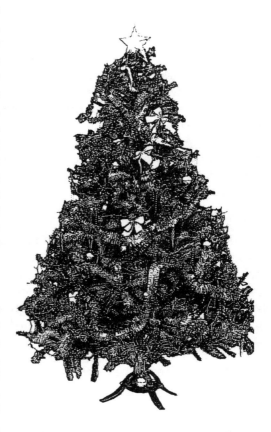

The words you use to describe yourself and the circumstances you are faced with can really increase the tension when you suffer an episode of stress, depression or anxiety. As you know, sufferers tend to focus on single, negative and catastrophic outcomes to their circumstances. In doing so, they use powerful words and expressions charged with frightening emotions. Being careful of the words and phrases you use to describe events you are faced with and to assign meanings to your life is a crucial skill.

W is for Work

Changes in attitudes to work and the way we now structure our working lives leads to a huge increase in stress in the workplace. Long working hours, heavy workload, pressure to meet targets and career progression are all placing enormous demands on individuals. As the pressure mounts, stress levels soar and this coupled with a lack of quality relaxation and leisure time and the demands of family life, is pushing many people to their limits. It is crucial to develop the skill of striking a balance between work and home life. Time spent with your loved ones, time spent enjoying hobbies, pastimes and socialising are equally as important as work is. Too much work will have consequences in all areas of your life so please be aware of the pressures too much work can bring and make time to relax and enjoy family and leisure time as well.

X is for Xmas

Christmas is supposed to be a lovely time of the year, a time for peace and goodwill, for feasting, for spending time with loved ones and of course, for giving and receiving gifts and presents! However, for many people the festive season can bring stress, depression and anxiety. Demands of shopping, wrapping presents, sending cards, preparing a sumptuous feast for the family, organising parties – all send stress levels soaring and can trigger anxiety. For people who have maybe lost a loved one or have separated from their partners or who live alone, Christmas can bring loneliness and sadness and descent into depression. Being organised is important. So plan well. Ensure everyone in the family is helping out and doing their share of the work. Remember, if everything does not go perfectly, it does not really matter. The skills that alleviate stress, depression and anxiety really do come into their own during the festive season and will ensure that all of the feelings, emotions, pressures and hard work do not lead to an episode of mental trauma.

Y is for YOU –

Self deprecation is the destructive self talk common to all sufferers of stress depression and anxiety. It is one of the worst things you can do to yourself. Putting yourself down at every opportunity, reminding yourself over and over again of your bad points and telling yourself that you're useless, boring, dull, incompetent and other mean things – is the definite way to lower your levels of confidence and self esteem. Please respect yourself. Never ever allow your mind to use self-deprecation against you. It is such a destructive and harmful practice.

Z is for Zero Hour

Zero Hour is defined in the Oxford English Dictionary as:-

> *"the specified time for an operation to begin"*

Stress, depression and anxiety can be beaten. You can develop the power to remove these dreadful problems out of your life once and for all. Make this the hour where you decide to start the fight back, to begin your operation on overcoming stress, depression and anxiety permanently. This is really important because until you reach the point where you are determined enough to take action to end the torment, stress, anxiety and depression will continue to spoil the happiness you deserve from life. Do not let this happen. Zero Hour is here.

Now that you have a better understanding of stress, and realise the proven very strong link it has with your Bipolar Disorder, it is time to start taking some definite steps to reduce the stress in your life and thereby reduce the symptoms of Bipolar Disorder. Here is a programme of nine steps that you should address immediately where appropriate.

STRESS REDUCTION STRATEGY

- Write down everything you have to do when you are feeling overwhelmed. Set a time frame, then mark what when you will accomplish. By divvying up your workload into manageable chunks, each with an allotted time, you will feel more relaxed about the work before you.

- Concentrate on one task at a time. Stressing about work you have not done yet only detracts from accomplishing the task at hand.

- Manage your energies wisely, prioritise your workload and put in less effort for low-priority jobs, and avoid expending energy on unimportant tasks.

- Delegate responsibility and get outside help if you feel overwhelmed. Employ a gardener or a babysitter for your child when you feel pressed for time.

- Reward yourself for accomplishing things. Acknowledge the work you put in and give yourself a pat on the back, instead of immediately rushing into the next task and creating more stress.

- Take small breaks during work. Visit a nearby café or take a quick walk, or allow yourself ten minutes to relax in your office: Close your eyes, clear your mind of work-related thoughts, visualise a pleasant landscape or holiday scene and relax your muscles.

- Exercise regularly to maintain your health and release stress, or take up a hobby. Set aside some quiet time to meditate and relax.

- Take a holiday. If indulging in a long holiday and staying away from work seems even more stressful, try taking several short breaks a year.

- Maintain your perspective by asking yourself, "Is the situation at hand really that serious that I should become stressed-out about it?"

Does this seem almost self-defeating? Do you feel that talk about more leisure, holidays and generally taking some quality time will mean that you will not have enough hours in the day to handle and manage the task that you do have already? Perhaps the tasks that at the moment you feel overwhelming you, the tasks that you feel require a thirty six hour day in order to accomplish them. The reality is totally different. The experience of most people is that when they begin to manage their lives better, and on a more even keel, they accomplish more than they would ever have dreamed possible. Here is an example from the world of athletics. It is by no means unusual for national and international competitive athletes to train seven days a week in order to attain the absolute peak of performance in their chosen sport.

Research was done to assess the impact of taking one rest day per week, and only training six days out of seven. The overwhelming conclusion was that athletes who did this performed better than their fellows who trained for seven days a week. Then the research was extended to look into a possible five day training cycle, with two full days off. The results were very surprising and showed that these athletes performed better still. The reality is that the athletes who were more relaxed about their training and took sufficient rest and time off work able to do far more

139

when it came to the day of racing than those who trained longer and harder.

In a similar way you will find that giving yourself time to recover, to rest and enjoy quality time, perhaps with your family and friends, will have a positive and dynamic impact on your performance when you are at work or doing whatever activities you normally spend your time doing.

Now it is time to take action. Copy or make your own Stress Reduction record and begin working on achieving the tasks suggested. As you achieve the task tick the box concerned and keep the weekly sheets so that you can keep an eye on your progress and make sure that you are working towards reducing your stress level.

Remember, the less stress, the less you will suffer from Bipolar Disorder symptoms

At the end of Chapter 7, as well as the stress reduction techniques and keeping a record, would you fill in another Mood Compass. As before, file it with your previous record sheets and try tol gauge how much progress you are making

Stress Reduction Record   Week ending ....

Tick the box for each activity you have achieved each day

Stress Reduction Activity	Sunday	Monday	Tuesday	Wednesday	Thursday	Friday	Saturday
1							
2							
3							
4							
5							
6							
7							
8							
9							

1. Write down everything you have to do when you're feeling overwhelmed. Set a time frame, then block out when you will accomplish what.

2 Concentrate on one task at a time. Stressing about work you haven't done yet only detracts from accomplishing the task at hand.

3 Manage your energies wisely, prioritize your workload and put in less effort for low-priority jobs, and avoid expending energy on unimportant tasks.

4 Delegate responsibility and get outside help if you feel overwhelmed. Hire a gardener for your lawn or a baby sitter for your child when you feel pressed for time.

5 Reward yourself for accomplishing things. Acknowledge the work you put in and give yourself a pat on the back, instead of immediately rushing into the next task and creating more stress.

6 Take small breaks during work. Visit a nearby café or take a quick walk, or allow yourself 10 minutes to relax in your office: Close your eyes, strip your mind of work-related thoughts, visualize a pleasant landscape or vacation scene and relax your muscles.

7 Exercise regularly to maintain your health and release stress, or take up a hobby. Set aside some quiet time to meditate and relax.

8 Give yourself vacations. If indulging in a long vacation (and staying away from work) seems even more stressful, try taking several short vacations per year.

9 Maintain your perspective by asking yourself, "Is the situation at hand really that serious that I should become stressed-out about it?

MENTAL REACTION

MIND

PHYSICAL REACTION

BODY

CHAPTER EIGHT

COGNITIVE BEHAVIOURAL THERAPY

"We found that people with depression who have increased activity in one area of the brain and decreased activity in another in response to emotional stimuli are more likely to respond to a specific treatment -- cognitive therapy."

Greg J. Siegle

CBT is a therapy that has emerged more recently as an extremely effective nondrug therapy for Bipolar sufferers, amongst others. Cognitive therapy helps the sufferer by assisting them to uncover and their thoughts and perceptions, which may have become distorted overtime and are causing them to suffer unduly. Before we look into the whole area of Cognitive Behavioural Therapy and examine how it works both in theory and in practice, let us remind ourselves of the symptoms of Bipolar Disorder that CBT is aiming to treat.

Mania:

A distinct period of abnormally that is persistently elevated, expansive or irritable mood.

- inflated self-esteem or grandiosity
- decreased need for sleep (e.g., feels rested after only three hours of sleep)
- more talkative than usual or pressure to keep talking
- flight of ideas or subjective experience that thoughts are racing; distractibility
- increase in goal-directed activity (either socially, at work or school, or sexually) or psychomotor agitation, especially activities that have a high potential for painful consequences (e.g., buying sprees, sexual indiscretions, or foolish business investments)

Depressive episode (symptoms are all, or most of the time; subjectively report or reported by others).

- pervasive depressed mood
- markedly diminished interest or pleasure in all, or almost all, activities
- significant weight loss when not dieting or weight gain
- insomnia or hypersomnia
- agitation
- fatigue or loss of energy nearly every day
- feelings of worthlessness or excessive or inappropriate guilt (which may be delusional)
- diminished ability to think or concentrate, or indecisiveness
- recurrent thoughts of death (not just fear of dying) or suicide

Notice that the whole issue of our thoughts, beliefs and the way we think and analyse situations is fundamental to the diagnosis of Bipolar Disorder. It is precisely these thoughts and beliefs that CBT aims to target. At least those thoughts and beliefs that are both incorrect and unhelpful. The theory of CBT was discovered and developed over thirty years ago. The idea is that your thoughts mediate between various stimuli, such as various events, together with a range of emotions. Is as you receive a stimulus, then you generate a thought, possibly some kind of judgement or evaluation of the stimulus that you have received. The stimulus gives rise to the thought which then becomes an emotion. In effect although the emotion is directly resulting from the stimulus there is the intermediate step of the thought which will in itself modify the combination of stimulus and the thought. This gives the resulting emotion or emotional response.

To make this a little clearer, let us take a simple example. John was unemployed and applied for a job. He was told that his application was unsuccessful. This negative response to his job application is the stimulus. He then feels that he was just not good enough to successfully get the job. This is the thought. The combination of the stimulus and the thought can then manifest itself as depression, this is the resultant emotion. Had John had a totally different thought about his failure to get the job he had applied for, the result would have been very different.

For example, following the negative response he assesses that there were a large number of applicants for the job and someone with possibly more experience or better qualifications than he had was judged to be more suited for that particular job. Had the vacancy be more suited to his experience and qualifications it was likely that he would have won the job. Therefore merely by altering the thought that he had as a response to the stimulus of the failed job application would then alter entirely the emotion that he felt, and instead of depression his resulting emotion may have been at worst a neutral emotion, and possibly a positive emotion of determination to keep looking for a job until something ceases to his skills and qualifications came up.

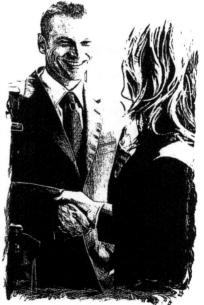

Cognitive and/or behavioural psychotherapies (CBP) are therefore psychological approaches based on scientific principles and which research has shown to be effective for a wide range of problems. Clients and therapists work together, once a therapeutic alliance has been formed, to identify and understand problems in terms of the relationship between thoughts, feelings and behaviour. The approach usually focuses on difficulties in the present, and relies on the therapist and client developing a shared view of the individual's problem. This then leads to identification of personalised, usually time-limited therapy goals and strategies which are continually monitored and evaluated. The treatments are inherently empowering in nature, the outcome being to focus on specific psychological and practical skills (e.g. in reflecting on and exploring the meaning attributed to events and situations and re-evaluation of those meanings) aimed at enabling the client to tackle their problems by harnessing their own resources.

If no severe co-morbid disorders (e.g. severe personality disorders) are present the therapy can be extremely effective, in both one to one and group based therapy sessions. Results are very promising, as up to 80% of patients show a significant improvement with appropriate therapy strategies. The main goal of this therapy is to identify and change inappropriate thoughts and patterns that underlie and perpetuate the course of the panic attacks. Very often a vicious cycle of dysfunctional thoughts (catastrophic depression and manic cycles) can be effectively treated by CBT, although in the severest of cases it is entirely likely that some form of medication will be required, at least in the early stages of treatment.

CBT offers strategies to help deal with the extremes of Bipolar Disorder and ways to cope with the situation, thus mitigating the worst of the symptoms. Sufferers are able to learn appropriate ways to face the manic and depressive stages of the disorder and, perhaps more importantly or equally importantly, to use CBT to have both an effective indicator of the onset of the mood extremes and to have strategies to deal with them.

Cognitive Behavioural therapy (CBT) is a symptom oriented therapy approach that combines psychoeducation with specific treatment intervention. The main components may include:-

- Psychoeducation = information
- self-monitoring of symptoms = prediction of the onset of symptoms
- breathing retraining/relaxation techniques = a response to the early warning of the onset of symptoms and a coping mechanism when the symptoms become severe
- cognitive restructuring to correct catastrophic misinterpretations of bodily and emotional sensations

At the beginning of each CBT treatment the therapist will try to explain the normal reactions of the body and symptoms related to Bipolar Disorder. The therapists will try to explain the treatment approaches and should also talk about the prognosis or possible problems of therapy. Psychoeducation usually includes help to identify early signs of relapse of anxiety symptoms and self-help options to cope with these situations.

One of the most effective help for patients with Bipolar symptoms is a diary or protocol of extreme attacks of mania and depression. To monitor the occurrence of symptoms, anxious cognitions and the consequences of changed behaviour (e.g. avoidance behaviour) is very important to get a rational description of the actual problem and to evaluate the treatment process. Patients are informed that this will help in the assessment of the frequency and nature of the onset of their symptoms and provide data regarding the relationship of these symptoms to various stimuli.

Cognitive restructuring techniques are used to identify and counter fear of bodily and emotional sensations. Most commonly, such thinking involves overestimation of the probability of a negative consequence and catastrophic thinking about the meaning of such sensations. Patients are encouraged to consider the evidence and to think of alternative possible outcomes following the experience of the bodily cue. Part of this process involves identifying the likely origin of the symptoms and/or any misinformation about the meaning of the sensations. The cognitive restructuring component of CBT is usually conducted by using a Socratic teaching method.

By means of these techniques is to take responsibility for one's emotions and therefore empower oneself to bring about the kind of change that is needed to reduce the symptoms of Bipolar Disorder and improve the quality of life. It is entirely possible to change the way we think, the way we feel and the way we act. Change can be made now and we can free ourselves from the behaviour patterns that are to some extent responsible for the extreme symptoms of Bipolar Disorder. We do not need to assume that nothing can be altered with regards to our behaviour. Everything is possible and indeed using the correct tools and techniques changed is certainly probable.

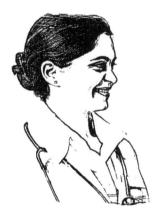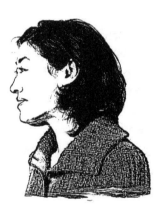

Cognitive Behavioural Therapy therefore examines the three-step process that leads to problematic thinking and the resultant behaviour. The three steps are stimulus, thought and emotion. CBT takes a logical and commonsense approach to thinking to help overcome the flawed thinking that has resulted in the manifestation of many of the problems we are suffering from now. The example of the man who was turned down for a job application is classic and shows how flawed thinking in a huge variety of situations can bring on wholly unwarranted and unnecessary negative responses and extreme symptoms of Bipolar Disorder. In essence it is a process of short-circuiting the three steps of stimulus, thought and emotion by interrupting the negative thought that he is an acquired and learned response with the thought that is more positive, more helpful and indeed more appropriate. This will then result in an emotion that is more balanced and indeed more positive than the negative emotion that is felt by Bipolar sufferers as well as sufferers of a range of other disorders such as anxiety and phobias.

Automatic thoughts are repetitive, automatic self-statements that we always say to ourselves in certain situations. They can be positive or negative. Psychological problems develop when our automatic thoughts are consistently negative. They are automatic, because they are not the result of an analysis of the problem, they are a "knee-jerk" reaction to specific situations.

For example, in social situations, do you always presume the other person dislikes you, or thinks you are stupid? When automatic thoughts control our emotional response to people, problems, and events, we ignore evidence that contradicts the automatic thought. If we cannot ignore it, we explain the evidence in terms of the automatic thought.

For example, if we talk to someone and they smile, they are really laughing at us, rather than being pleased to see us. The automatic thoughts create an expectancy of something negative.

Since many things in life are vague, and can be interpreted in many ways, we learn how to negatively evaluate the world, so it agrees with our negative automatic thoughts. Psychologists help you to identify your negative automatic thoughts, and how to develop positive challenges to those negative ideas.

CBT will examine and re-evaluate the kind of thoughts that you have about yourself, about your skills, your achievements, your abilities and even your physical appearance and behaviour. That is not a question of suddenly reinventing yourself as a very different and perhaps very superior person, physically, socially and emotionally. Rather it is a process of examining the flawed thinking that has given the lie to so many things about ourselves and has resulted in depressive and manic behaviour.

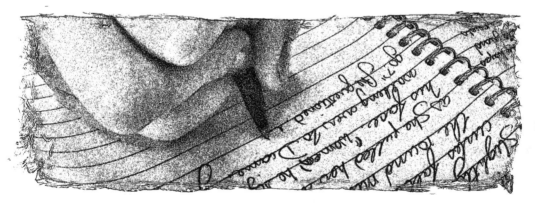

It is perhaps difficult to simply envisage exactly what is a "thought". In fact there are two distinct types of thought which we will need to examine.

On the one hand there are inferences. An inference is an assumption that you make about certain facts occur during your life. For example if you are driving a car and an old friend who was a very experienced driver suddenly advises you on that you are going too fast, you could infer from this that they are criticising your driving and possibly suggesting that you are a reckless driver. An alternative thought it could be that the friend is aware that perhaps you have been distracted by something and it is concerned that you do not get a ticket for speeding. Clearly leads to inferences would be totally opposite. In the first case it is a negative inference and in the second case a positive influence, showing that your friend is very concerned for your welfare and he is prepared to make an effort to help you to avoid an unpleasant situation.

The first thought that of criticism, could then easily lead to the beginnings of irritation and possibly rage, then leading to a measure of depression that "my friends don't like me". CBT is aimed at helping you to make much more helpful and realistic responses to stimuli such as the second response, i.e. a calm and happy feeling that your friend is sufficiently caring and concerned about you to make the effort to help you avoid a speeding ticket.

The other set of thoughts that we have about ourselves evaluative thoughts, which can be described as beliefs. And evaluative thought means that we have made a judgement, about ourselves or about others or, about some situation that exists in the world. These evaluative thoughts, frequently known as beliefs, building blocks in the process of forming feelings and behaviour is about ourselves that are either negative or positive. Bipolar Disorder patients can therefore use CBT skills to identify and respond to negative core beliefs, such as "Nobody cares about me" or "I am incompetent". Addressing these beliefs is essential when delivering or undertaking CBT because they are likely to intensify the depressive episodes. Through implementing CBT, patients can also develop anxiety-management strategies and reduce symptoms of depression.

The cognitive component in the cognitive behavioural psychotherapies refers to how people think about and create meaning about situations, symptoms and events in their lives and develop beliefs about themselves, others and the world. Cognitive therapy uses techniques to help people become more aware of how they reason, and the kinds of automatic thought that spring to mind and give meaning to things.

Cognitive interventions use a style of questioning to probe for peoples' meanings and use this to stimulate alternative viewpoints or ideas. This is called "guided discovery", and involves exploring and reflecting on the style of reasoning and thinking, and possibilities to think differently and more helpfully. On the basis of these alternatives people carry out behavioural experiments to test out the accuracy of these alternatives, and thus adopt new ways of perceiving and acting. Overall the intention is to move away from more extreme and unhelpful ways of seeing things to more helpful and balanced conclusions. The behavioural component in the cognitive behavioural psychotherapies refers to the way in which people respond when distressed. Responses such as avoidance, reduced activity and unhelpful behaviours can act to keep the problems going or worsen how the person feels. CBT practitioners aim to help the person feel safe enough to gradually test out their assumptions and fears and change their behaviours. For example this might include helping people to gradually face feared or avoided situations as a means to reducing anxiety and learning new behavioural skills to tackle problems. Importantly the cognitive and behavioural psychotherapies aim to directly target distressing symptoms, reduce distress, re-evaluate thinking and promote helpful behavioural responses by offering problem-focussed skills-based treatment interventions.

Bipolar Response Record Chart

	Stimulus – Event etc.	My response emotion	Was this appropriate?	Better, Modified Response Emotion	Resulting emotion
Sunday					
Monday					
Tuesday					
Wednesday					
Thursday					
Friday					
Saturday					

This is an example of a simple chart or journal that you can keep in order that as you go through each day you can record your responses, i.e. thoughts, to the various stimuli that you come across. In this way you will be able to monitor those occasions when you feel that you response to stimuli in a way that is both incorrect and unhelpful, reconsider your response and keep a written record of a healthier and more positive response for when this stimulus occurs in the future.

Some of the key components of CBT are:-

- the main focus is on the here-and-now
- the main goal is to help you to bring about the positive change you desire
- there is a focus on learning new skills which empower you
- the aim is to bring about positive practical lasting change in every day living
- problem solving is a key part of therapy
- therapy is extremely transparent and all rationale is clearly explained
- the therapist's role is that of teacher in imparting new skills to you
- The therapist works with you in a collaborative relationship
- you are fully involved in all decisions
- problems and strategies are worked out and planned together
- the success of therapy is dependent on your engagement and active participation in the process of change

CBT can help you to make sense of overwhelming problems by breaking them down into smaller parts. This makes it easier to see how they are connected and how they affect you. CBT aims to get you to a point where you can "do it yourself", and work out your own ways of tackling these problems by breaking the cycle of distress.

Here is a typical story of one person's approach to Cognitive Behavioural Therapy.

"Social anxiety has affected me since I was in school. While it was triggered initially by a traumatic experience, it is something that runs in the family and I certainly had a predisposition for.

Some examples of how it manifested itself over the years:-

- avoiding certain types of social situations and friends
- avoiding public speaking
- avoiding the opposite sex completely
- hiding in the library during lunchtime
- the thought of just walking down certain hallways at school terrified me,
- fear of being around large groups of people
- fear and avoidance of going to parties or social gatherings

My social anxiety became severe and I dropped out of college after semester. That's when I started to get uncomfortable just leaving my apartment and hit "the bottom" so to speak. Through treatment with group Cognitive Behavioural Therapy (CBT) and medication I've been able to live the balanced life that I value and form healthy friendships and relationships. CBT was effective for learning to think, act and feel differently in social situations.

The cognititve treatment included techniques for disrupting, stopping and later turning around negative thoughts, relaxation techniques, dealing with setbacks, slow talk to control anxiety, deserving statements, among other things.

The behavioural portion includes strategy for creating and following an anxiety hierarchy, which involves creating an ordered list of things that cause you anxiety and slowly working your way up and doing them while trying to maintain a reasonable level of anxiety using the cognitive techniques learned.

At first it didn't feel I I was getting any better or making any progress, but I kept at it day in and day out (missing days on occasion and trying not to feel too guilty about it) and with time I started to notice small changes in how negatively I was viewing myself, others and social situations, along with lower levels of anxiety in social situations.

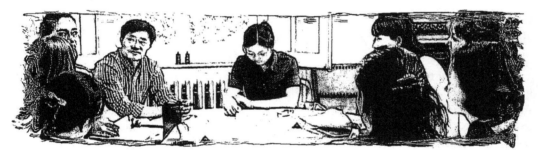

The big progress came later when I participated in a twenty week group session. The group leader and the other participants were very supportive.

Ultimately, the real benefits of the cognitive therapy and behavioural exercises, on my own and with the group, took months to materialise. It was hard work, took persistence and courage, and there were setbacks, but my life took a turn down a new path as a result. "

Sometimes a depressed person may accurately identify a skill deficit. "I'm not good at telling people what I want from them." This is usually coupled with negative self-evaluation, "therefore, it's my fault that I didn't get what I want." However, in depression, the person assumes that they cannot learn how to do what is necessary to achieve a better outcome. The depressed person believes they cannot learn how to act differently. Accurate identification of social skill deficits complicates depression, because it provides a reality base for the other irrational and exaggerated negative perceptions of the depressed person. If the skill deficit is real, then the depressed person assumes that all of the other negative self-assessments must be real too.

Further, when depressed, a person is more likely to identify negative characteristics of self, and less likely to see the positive.

The result is a long list of:-

- "things I cannot do "
- "tasks I'm no good at"
- "mistakes I've made"

Psychologists help depressed persons identify their social skill deficits, and also help them develop a plan to improve those skills. This part of cognitive therapy is more behavioural, as the psychologist teaches the depressed person how to manage their life problems better.

When depressed, a person will focus on minor negative aspects of what was otherwise a positive life experience. For example, after a holiday at the beach, the depressed person will remember the one day it rained, rather than the six days of sunshine. If anything goes wrong, the depressed person evaluates the entire experience as a failure, or as a negative life experience. As a result, memories are almost always negative. This is reflective of unrealistic expectations. Nothing in life ever works out just as you want. If we expect perfection, we will always be disappointed. Psychologists help you to develop realistic expectations about life, and help you determine what you need versus what you want. After all, most of the things that fail to work out are little things. And even when important problems develop, we can either resolve the problem, regroup, recover and start again, with hope for a better future. In depression, the hope is missing.

Psychological treatment of depression (psychotherapy) can assist the depressed individual in several ways. First, supportive counselling helps ease the pain of depression, and addresses the feelings of hopelessness that accompany depression. Second, cognitive therapy changes the pessimistic ideas, unrealistic expectations and overly critical self-evaluations that create depression and sustain it. Cognitive therapy helps the depressed person recognise which life problems are critical and which are minor. It also helps him/her to develop positive life goals, and a more positive self-assessment. Third, problem solving therapy changes the areas of the person's life that are creating significant stress, and contributing to the depression. This may require behavioural therapy to develop better coping skills, or interpersonal therapy, to assist in solving relationship problems.

At first glance, this may seem like several different therapies being used to treat depression. However, all of these interventions are used as part of a cognitive treatment approach. Some psychologists use the phrase, Cognitive Behavioural Therapy and others simply call this approach, cognitive therapy. In practice, both cognitive and behavioural techniques are used together.

Once upon a time, behaviour therapy did not pay any attention to cognitions, such as perceptions, evaluations or expectations. Behaviour therapy only studied behaviour that could be observed and measured. But, psychology is a science, studying human thoughts, emotions and behaviour. Scientific research has found that perceptions, expectations, values, attitudes, personal evaluations of self and others, fears, desires, etc. are all human experiences that affect behaviour. Also, our behaviour, and the behaviour of others, affects all of those cognitive experiences as well.

Thus, cognitive and behavioural experiences are intertwined, and must be studied, changed or eliminated, as an interactive pair.

Many people think that cognitive therapy is a relatively recent development in psychotherapy. However, Albert Ellis published, Reason and Emotion in Psychotherapy in 1962, and Aaron Beck wrote about, The Self Concept in Depression with D. Stein in 1960. To some extent, most or all of the psychodynamic and psychoanalytic theories of depression can be described as having cognitive components.

For example, Freud, in Mourning and Melancholia, published in 1917, suggests that melancholia (depression) can occur in response to an imaginary or perceived loss, and that self-critical aspects of the ego are responsible in part for depression.

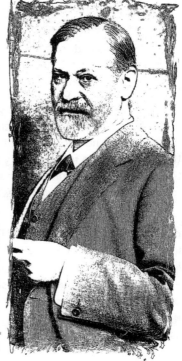

The main difference between these psychodynamic therapies and cognitive therapies lies in the motivational assumptions made by the therapists, and the techniques used to effect change. Psychodynamic theories presume that the maladaptive cognitions arise from specific internal needs (such as the need for affection, acceptance, sexual gratification, etc.), or from unresolved developmental conflicts from childhood. The cognitive therapists presume that the maladaptive cognitions may arise from faulty social learning, or from a lack of experiences that would allow adaptive learning (such as the development of coping skills) to occur, or from dysfunctional family experiences, or from traumatic events, etc. In other words, psychologists using a cognitive therapy approach recognise that psychological problems such as depression can develop from a variety of life experiences, depending on the individual.

In the 1970s, many psychologists began writing about cognitive aspects of depression, identifying different cognitive components that affected depression, and developing cognitive interventions to treat depression. From this base of theory and research came evidence that cognitive therapy was an effective, and perhaps is the most effective, intervention strategy for treating depression. Since the 1970s, the use of cognitive therapy with depression has increased tremendously, and the number of psychologists using cognitive therapy approaches for the treatment of all psychological problems has also grown. As a result, it appears that cognitive therapy has recently appeared on the scene, in only the past twenty years. But, all psychotherapy has cognitive components. One of the major differences between cognitive therapy and other therapy approaches is the treatment interventions used to change human cognitive experiences.

Cognitive Factors in Depression

- self-evaluation
- identification of skill deficits
- evaluation of life experiences
- self-talk
- automatic thoughts
- irrational ideas and beliefs
- over generalising
- cognitive distortions
- pessimistic thinking

Self-evaluation is a process that is ongoing. We evaluate how we are managing life tasks and whether we are doing what we should, saying what we should, or acting the way we should. In depression, self-evaluation is generally negative and critical. When a mistake occurs, we think, "I messed up. I'm no good at anything. It's my fault things went wrong". When someone is depressed, they tend to take responsibility for everything that goes wrong, and to give others credit for things that turn out fine. Psychologists assume that self-evaluation in depressed individuals is too critical, and feeds low self-esteem and a sense of failure.

Sometimes a depressed person may accurately identify a skill deficit. "I'm not good at telling people what I want from them." This is usually coupled with negative self-evaluation. "Therefore, it's my fault that I didn't get what I want." However, in depression, the person assumes they cannot learn how to do what is necessary to achieve a better outcome or learn how to act differently. Accurate identification of social skill deficits complicates depression, because it provides a reality base for the other irrational and exaggerated negative perceptions of the depressed person. If the skill deficit is real, then the depressed person assumes that all of the other negative self-assessments must be real too. Further when depressed, a person is more likely to identify negative characteristics of self, and less likely to see the positive.

The result is a long list of the –

- "things I cannot do"
- "tasks I'm no good at"
- "mistakes I've made"

Psychologists help depressed persons identify their social skill deficits, and also to develop a plan to improve those skills. This part of cognitive therapy is more behavioural, as the psychologist teaches the depressed person how to manage their life problems better.

When depressed a person will focus on minor negative aspects of what was otherwise a positive life experience. If anything goes wrong, the depressed person evaluates the entire experience as a failure, or as a negative life experience. As a result, memories are almost always negative. This is reflective of unrealistic expectations. Nothing in life ever works out just as you want. If we expect perfection, we will always be disappointed. Psychologists help you to develop realistic expectations about life, and help you determine what you need versus what you want. After all, most of the things that do not work out are little things. And even when important problems develop, we can resolve the problem, recover or start again, with hope for a better future.

Self-talk is a way of describing all the things we say to ourselves all day long as we confront obstacles, make decisions, and resolve problems. Self-talk is not talking to yourself in a literal sense, although it sometimes does involve talking out loud (depending on the person). There is a myth, that when you talk to yourself, it is a sign of craziness or mental illness. That idea stems from the voices or auditory hallucinations experienced in severe forms of mental illness, such as Schizophrenia. When a person hears voices, they think someone else talking to them. The self-talk we are describing here is not like that at all. We all engage in self-talk. Usually it is part of our thinking process, or what we call stream of consciousness.

As we are presented with problems or decisions, we might think-

- "Okay, how do I handle this?"
- "This looks like it is difficult, I better ask for help."
- "I know how to fix this!"

Self-talk is not bad, wrong or a sign of psychological problems. It is normal. But, negative self-talk prevents us from solving problems and can contribute to a variety of psychological problems, including depression.

When faced with a problem, if our self-talk is negative, it can immobilise us –

- "I can't do this, I'm just going to foul it up again"
- "I'll probably get fired after they see how incompetent I am."

Psychologists help depressed individuals identify negative self-talk, and also teach them how to challenge these negative statements and replace them with positive self-talk.

Automatic thoughts are repetitive, automatic self-statements that we always say to ourselves in certain situations. They can be positive or negative. Psychological problems develop when our automatic thoughts are consistently negative. They are automatic, because they are not the result of an analysis of the problem, they are a reaction to specific situations. For example, in social situations, do you always presume the other person dislikes you, or thinks you are stupid? When automatic thoughts control our emotional response to people, problems and events, we ignore evidence that contradicts the automatic thought. If we cannot ignore it, we explain the evidence in terms of the automatic thought.

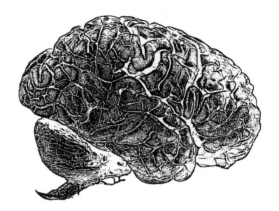

For example, if we talk to someone and they smile, they are really laughing at us, rather than being pleased to see us. The automatic thoughts create an expectancy of something negative. Since many things in life are vague, and can be interpreted in many ways, we learn how to negatively evaluate the world, so it agrees with our negative automatic thoughts. Psychologists help you to identify your negative automatic thoughts, and how to develop positive challenges to those negative ideas.

Albert Ellis first presented the idea that irrational beliefs are at the core of most psychological problems. We could also call these beliefs unrealistic, incorrect or maladaptive. Psychologists have also suggested that these ideas are irrational because they are not logical, or are based on false assumptions. Some examples of irrational beliefs:

- I cannot be happy unless everyone likes me.
- If I do what is expected of me, my life will be wonderful.
- Bad things don't happen to good people.
- Good things don't happen to bad people.
- In the end, bad people will always get punished.
- If I am intelligent (or work hard), I will be successful.

What makes these ideas irrational is the belief that they are always correct. Yes, working hard will increase your chances for success, but success is not guaranteed. There are times when we do everything right and we still do not get what we want. For some people this leads to the conclusion that they are lazy, no good, incompetent or weak. The result is a loss of self-esteem and sometimes depression. Psychologists help you to identify your irrational ideas, and also how to evaluate which ideas are irrational and which are not. Finally, the ideas need to be changed to reflect the real world.

Catastrophising is a negative overgeneralisation. It is "making a mountain out of a mole hill!"

For example:-

- One person at work does not like you, and tells you, so you know it's not mistaken judgment. You then assume no one at work likes you, or you assume that you must be a terrible person if he/she does not like you.

- You make a small mistake on a project and assume that you will be fired when the boss finds out.
- You try your hand at a new hobby and it does not turn out well. You conclude, "I'm no good at anything."

We all make mistakes. If you overgeneralise one, or even a few mistakes, to the conclusion that you are bad, incompetent or useless, you might become depressed. Psychologists help you identify and change negative overgeneralisations.

Cognitive distortions are another way of describing the irrational ideas, overgeneralising of simple mistakes, or developing false assumptions about what other people think about or expect from us. We are distorting reality by the way we are evaluating a situation. The concept of cognitive distortion highlights the importance of perceptions, assumptions and judgments in coping with the world. Psychologists help us determine what evaluations are distortions by providing objective feedback about our evaluations of the world, and by teaching us how to change the way we perceive problems.

Pessimistic thinking does not cause depression, but it appears to be easier to become depressed if you tend to view the world with considerable pessimism. After all, pessimism is a tendency to think that things will not work out as you wish and that you will not get what you want. Pessimism feeds the negative cognitive distortions and self-talk. On the other hand, optimism appears to create some protection from depression.

Hopelessness is a central feature of depression, along with helplessness. If you view your world as bad, filled with problems and don't think you can do anything about the problems, you will feel helpless. If you believe your life will not improve, if you think the future is bleak, then you will begin to feel hopeless. Pessimism encourages these negative assessments of your life. Optimism prevents you from reaching those conclusions. In fact, psychologists have researched ways to learn how to be more optimistic, as a way of fighting depression.

The crux of CBT treatment involves Cognitive restructuring, which enables patients to identify cognitive distortions, and to change these negative cognitive responses into more positive, realistic responses. Rehearsal of rational responses will allow core beliefs to be identified and challenged more easily.

Core beliefs following a traumatic experience typically include such beliefs as:-

- "The world is unsafe"
- "I cannot be well"
- "I am a coward"

Goal-setting, problem solving and relaxation are all important parts of Cognitive Behavioural Therapy for Bipolar sufferers. At the end of Chapter 8 you should have a good understanding of what CBT involves and how much it could mean to you.

TASKS

1. Firstly, you have the Bipolar Response Records Chart to work with and if you have not already done so, you should begin using this chart now.

2. Secondly, you need to identify goals that are important for you to achieve, or at least to aim at. Remember, completing all of your goals is not as essential or important as actually making efforts to achieve them. Once you have begun to make an effort you have won a critical battle in your fight against Bipolar Disorder. If you continue to make similar efforts they will build upon each other until such time as you begin to find the mitigation or indeed disappearance of many of your symptoms. Keep a simple list of goals and each time you achieve something towards one of them, put a tick against that goal. The ticks will soon build up, as will your optimism and self-esteem as a result. It is entirely likely that you will benefit from a CBT group. One goal could be to locate such a group and at least go along to one or two meetings to see what benefit it could be to you.

3. Thirdly, fill in another Mood Compass Chart and keep with your others. Are you progressing in your battle against bipolar disorder? The answer is an emphatic yes. You have identified the problem, faced up to it and are taking steps to resolve it. If you keep going, as no doubt you will, you will experience a happier, more fulfilled and positive life.

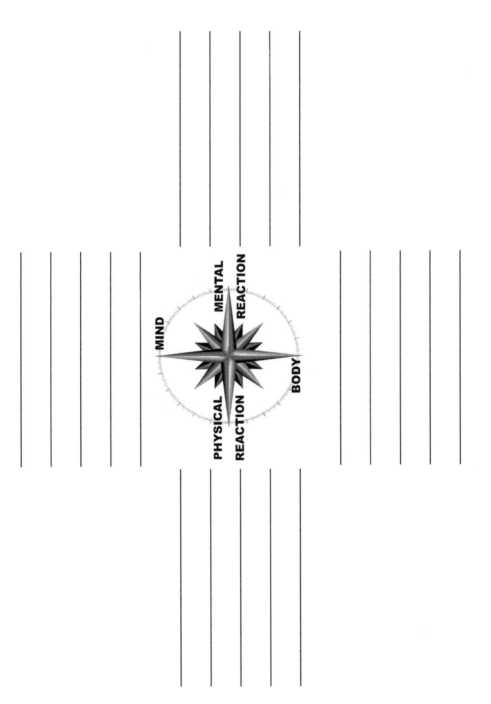

CHAPTER NINE

MEDITATION AND MINDFULNESS

"Peace can be reached through meditation on the knowledge which dreams give. Peace can also be reached through concentration upon that which is dearest to the heart."

Patanjali

In Chapter 9 we will be examining the very alternative treatments of meditation and mindfulness. Although this may conjure up images of Asian gurus in saffron robes with long flowing beards, the idea of using mindfulness meditation is one that goes back into the depths of history. The Buddhist religion teaches meditation and mindfulness as a powerful and effective path to calmness and relief from a range of emotional and mental traumas. The evidence suggests that whilst this may not stand as a complete and independent treatment or cure for Bipolar Disorder, it is still a very valuable part of the range of therapies on offer and should definitely be tried by anyone suffering from Bipolar Disorder.

Buddhists say that over 2500 years ago Buddha provided guidance on establishing mindfulness. Right mindfulness involves bringing one's awareness to focus on experience within the mind at the present moment (from the past, the future or some disconnected train of thought). By paying close attention to the present experience, practitioners begin to see both inner and outer aspects of reality as aspects of the mind. Internally, one sees that the mind is continually full of chattering with commentary or judgement. By noticing that the mind is continually making commentary, one has the ability to carefully observe those thoughts, seeing them for what they are without aversion or judgment. Those practicing mindfulness realise that thoughts are just thoughts. One is free to release a thought when one realises that the thought may not be concrete reality or absolute truth. Thus, one is free to observe life without getting caught in the commentary. Many voices or messages may speak to one within the vocal (discursive) mind. It is important to be aware that the messages one hears during thinking are simply discursive habits.

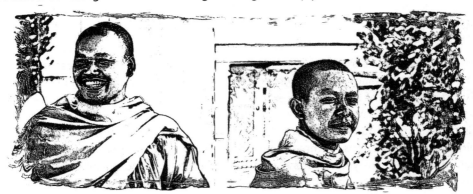

Mindfulness meditation is moment to moment awareness. It is being fully awake. It involves being here for the moments of our lives, without striving or judging. You will have felt it.

Let us explore one of those times now. Remember doing something you really, really enjoyed. Stop reading this and close your eyes and take a few moments to remember that time right now. How did you feel as you recalled it? Did you notice there was little room left for distracting thoughts or feelings? Bringing our full attention into anything is mindfulness. You step fully into the moment. There is a sense of completeness. These are the moments of our lives when we feel most at home.

Mindfulness involves a formal practice and an informal practice. In formal practice we take time for sitting meditation or mindful movement practices like walking meditation or yoga or chi gong. Informal practice is a way of life in which we meditate as we do what we do. It involves being present in the moments of our lives. As one Las Vegas casino warned, "YOU MUST BE PRESENT TO WIN". That's it! You must be present to love, experience peace, joy or contentment. When you are here you can have the experience of your life. Mindfulness involves being in each moment as it is without judgment or striving and having a kind of releasement towards things. It is a relaxed state of awareness that observes both your inner world of thoughts, feelings and sensations, and the outer world of constantly changing phenomena without trying to control anything.

The Mindfulness meditation technique is unique. But it's extremely effective, in fact a great way to bring yourself back to whatever you want to focus on. This meditation is very easy to learn and fun to practice. Remember that this meditation is intended to bring you to the present moment. You want to remain in the here and now as long as possible. If you find your mind drifting onto other matters in your life, simply bring your attention back to your body. Just pick up where you left off. We will look into how to get into mindfulness meditation at the end of the chapter, so do not be concerned at this stage, it is somewhat strange for the beginner to understand at first.

You should be aware that there are two stages to the process, both meditation and mindfulness. Concentrative meditation focuses the attention on the breath, an image or a sound (mantra), in order to still the mind and allow a greater awareness and clarity to emerge. This is like a zoom lens in a camera, we narrow our focus to a selected field.

The simplest form of concentrative meditation is to sit quietly and focus the attention on the breath. Yoga and meditation practitioners believe that there is a direct correlation between one's breath and one's state of the mind. For example, when a person is anxious, frightened, agitated or distracted, the breath will tend to be shallow, rapid and uneven. On the other hand when the mind is calm, focused and composed, the breath will tend to be slow, deep and regular. Focusing the mind on the continuous rhythm of inhalation and exhalation provides a natural object of meditation. As you focus your awareness on the breath, your mind becomes absorbed in the rhythm of inhalation and exhalation. As a result, your breathing will become slower and deeper, and the mind becomes more tranquil and aware.

The second component of this form of therapy is mindfulness. Mindfulness meditation involves opening the attention to become aware of the continuously passing parade of sensations and feelings, images, thoughts, sounds, smells and so forth without becoming involved in thinking about them. The person sits quietly and simply witnesses whatever goes through the mind, not reacting or becoming involved with thoughts, memories, worries or images. This helps to gain a more calm, clear and non-reactive state of mind. Mindfulness meditation can be likened to a wide-angle lens. Instead of narrowing your sight to a selected field as in concentrative meditation, here you will be aware of the entire field.

You may ask does this form of therapy work, and will it work for me? The answer for most people is a clear and emphatic yes! Studies have shown that meditation (in particular, research on Transcendental Meditation, a popular form of meditation practiced in the West for the past thirty years), can bring about a healthy state of relaxation. This is caused by a generalised reduction in multiple physiological and biochemical markers, such as decreased heart rate, decreased respiration rate, decreased plasma cortisol (a major stress hormone), decreased pulse rate, and increased EEG (electroencephalogram) alpha, a brain wave associated with relaxation. Research conducted by R. Keith Wallace at U.C.L.A. on Transcendental Meditation(TM), revealed that during meditation the body gains a state of profound rest. At the same time, the brain and mind become more alert, indicating a state of restful alertness. Studies show that after TM reactions are faster, creativity greater and comprehension broader.

A laboratory study of practitioners of Maharishi Mahesh Yogi's Transcendental Meditation, carried out by Benson and Wallace at Harvard Medical School towards the end of the 1960s, provided the first detailed knowledge of the many physiological changes associated with meditation. Some of the meditators, whose ages ranged from seventeen to forty-one, had been meditating only a few weeks. Others had for several years. All recorded changes associated with deep relaxation. The fall in metabolic rate was the most striking discovery. This was indicated by a dramatic drop in oxygen consumption within a few minutes of starting meditation. Consumption fell by up to 20% below the normal level, below that experienced even in deep sleep. Meditators took on average two breaths less and one litre less air per minute. The meditators' heart rate was several beats less per minute.

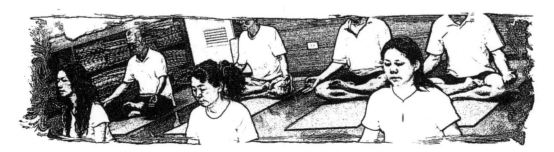

During meditation, blood pressure stayed at low levels, but fell markedly in persons starting meditation with abnormally high levels. The meditators' skin resistance to an electrical current was measured. A fall in skin resistance is characteristic of anxiety and tension states. A rise indicates increased muscle relaxation. The finding was that though meditation is primarily a mental technique, it soon brings significantly improved muscle relaxation. Meditation reduces activity in the nervous system. The parasympathetic branch of the autonomic or involuntary nervous system predominates. This is the branch responsible for calming us.

During anxiety and tension states there is a rise in the level of lactate in the blood. Lactate is a substance produced by metabolism in the skeletal muscles. During meditation blood lactate levels decreased at a rate four times faster than the rate of decrease in non-meditators resting lying on their backs or in the meditators themselves in pre-meditation resting.

The likely reason for the dramatic reduction in lactate production by meditators was indicated when further studies of meditators showed an increased blood flow during. Benson and Wallace found that there was a 32% increase in forearm blood flow. Lactate production in the body is mainly in skeletal muscle tissue; during meditation the faster circulation brings a faster delivery of oxygen to the muscles and less lactate is produced.

The two investigators summed up the state produced by their meditating subjects as wakeful and hypometabolic. The physiological changes were different in many ways from those found in sleeping people or those in hypnotic trance states. Meditation, they said, produces a complex of responses that marks a highly relaxed state. Moreover, the pattern of changes they observed in meditators suggested an integrated response, mediated by the central nervous system.

Taoists believe that the mind of emotions is governed by the fire energy of the heart. When your emotions are not controlled the fire energy of the heart flares upwards, wastefully burning up energy and clouding the mind. The mind of intent, or willpower, is controlled by the water energy of the kidneys. When unattended, the water energy flows down and out through the sexual organs, depleting essence and energy and weakening the spirit. Taoists believe that when you are sitting still doing nothing, as in meditation, the flow of fire and water are reversed: Water energy from the kidneys and sacrum is drawn up to the head via the central and governing channels, while emotional fire energy from the heart is drawn down into the Lower Elixir Field in the abdomen. There it is refined and transformed and enters general circulation through the energy channels. On the spiritual/mental level, this internal energy alchemy enables the mind of intent (water) to exert a calming, cooling, controlling influence over the mind of emotion (fire).

Let us begin looking at mindfulness meditation at a more practical level. There is no need to worry about having to turn into a Buddhist monk or nun to make a success of this. Western medicine has adopted the practice of meditation as a treatment therapy for a range of emotional challenges for several decades. The practice of mindfulness is also fast becoming an accepted therapy.

To practice body mindfulness meditation, one uses the breath as the way to connect and go into the body. With each breath, you notice what physical sensations there are. Each breath conditions the body, bringing oxygen to every cell in the body. Notice the way the breath feeds each and every part of you. There is an amazing connection between mindfulness and breath. The breath is an instrument for bringing about mindfulness to the body in a powerful way. It takes you to a place where you can make contact with your body without preference or hesitation.

Breath is not will but technique. Will is one's initial motive for cultivating spiritual goals and discipline. There is nothing wrong with having a desire for enlightenment. At same time, it is not sufficient to have that unless we practice meditative techniques. Just having will might turn one into divine frustration, since there will not be any transformative progress. It is like having fantasies about going to Tibet or some exotic country, but do nothing about it. Breath allows you to connect with yourself in a deeper way. The moment you focus on the breath, you'll begin to feel every aspect of your body, even at a cellular level.

Our body is multi dimensional, it is more then flesh and bone. It is a galaxy in its own way. Our body has all these cellular levels, each of them have a complete organism. Modern science describes that every cell in our body has some kind of intelligence and function. First of all, it is common understanding that without body, there is no way one can survive. The more we connect with our body, the more we are alive. Our usual tendency is to identify with thought and emotion. When we do that, we get stuck with them the way a car gets stuck in a ditch. That is the place where we repeat the same habitual patterns over and over again. In someway, we are not completely alive in each moment as long as we are not free from our habit. Our internal habits prevent us from connecting with our body.

Without being fully alive, there is no way we can go any further on the spiritual path. If we truly desire enlightenment, we have to learn how to be alive completely. When you are fully alive you are free from all internal conflicts, because you are in contact with reality. Our body is a doorway to connect with every momentary reality. Our body is not a separate entity from us. When we get stuck with our thoughts, fantasy and memory, we are in mental realms where everything is distorted. Meditation is not about leaving this body and playing with one's mind. When we are too much in a mental realm, we become so disconnected from everything and we no longer experience the wonder and freshness of every moment. Breathing is again a very powerful meditative tool. Along side that physical movement can be very helpful.

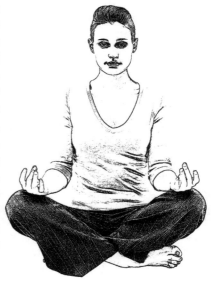

Here are some instructions for body mindfulness meditation:

- After doing physical movement, sit in the lotus position. Straighten your body and relax.

- First breathe gently for quite a while, while you breathe observe the breath as usual. Now and then breathe fast and actively.

- Make sure that when you breathe, you breathe all the way to belly, this is quite important. You'll experience the centeredness and the vitality of life. In Tibetan, it is called "bumtho" meaning vase belly.

- All the way through, let yourself observe the body. Deepen your awareness. Be aware of every bodily sensation. See that the body is changing in every moment. See it as quite different than how we see it most of the time. See the body as no longer this separated entity. You can experience there is no boundary between you and your body. Even the concepts of body will disappear. There will be only an experience of the body.

- Remember, do not ignore any sensation of body, even the subtle ones.

For most practitioners, mindfulness is the "same old, same old meditation". Of course, it came directly from Buddha two thousand years ago. In actuality what Buddha taught was a system or way of developing mindfulness, but mindfulness is not anyone's creation, not even the Buddha's. It is inherent in each and every one of us, whether or not one has done meditation. Sometimes it requires that we use meditative techniques and structures just for the purpose of igniting the amazing ability, which lies latent in each of us.

The paradox about mindfulness is that when you become very ambitious about cultivating it, this becomes an obstacle. It pushes meditation away instead of bringing it about. In some ways, it has nothing to do with how much you know about it and how many disciplines you have practiced. Its natural cultivation has to do with whether or not you get the idea. When we enter into a meditative state, we are entering into the realm of pure consciousness in which all our concepts are gone. There is only one meditation, it is a way of being in the moment and aware of everything around us. When we are fully in our body, we are already in the meditative state. It is much easier to practice those pseudo meditations than just being in the body.

While practicing body mindfulness, first one focuses on the belly where vitality is. Breathe all the way there. Awareness of that space will occur. Slowly, one can expand one's awareness throughout the body. Do not apply any other complicated method unless one does not know how to get the awareness. You may begin having a sense of bliss or rapture. Learn not to attach to them, let them pass by. This is a form of primal meditation in which we use our vitality for becoming aware of everything.

One can hide from facing reality now and then, but eventually no matter how strong your avoidance tactics are, you have to face the inevitability of your life situation. We do not know what is going to happen tomorrow. We could win the lottery or we could die by tomorrow. There is no way we can predict our future, even in the next moment. When we face those realities, we might not be ready for them. That is when we could completely fall apart. If we cannot find another easy way to escape, as we may have in the past, we might have to experience our emotions like a volcanic eruption. It is very easy to be lost in that emotional eruption. It is like being a child fighting amongst tigers.

The very reason we avoid our feelings and emotions is because we experience them as painful and sorrowful due to our attachment to them. We attach to our emotions by perceiving them as pleasant or unpleasant. We do that because we have such dualistic perception toward conditions as being either good or bad. This perception is so infantile and ignorant. We humans tend to conceptualise things based on our hopes and fears. With this perception toward reality, we will never be able to free ourselves from resistance and craving. To free ourselves, we must go beyond this fundamental perception of good and bad, life and death.

Connecting with one's emotions is a direct way of facing reality. We have suppressed and over-accumulated a great many past emotions because feeling them seems so painful, although they have nothing to do with reality. It is only a belief system. This moment is the time to explore them. Remember the saying, "now or never". You might feel grief about your lost friend that you had not fully processed. You might have a wound that goes back sometime ago, but did not have the tolerance to face.

When you truly allow yourself to reveal your old and long-held emotions, there will be awakening, an opening experience. That is when you are undertaking an inner journey in the moment in which you a re going to find liberation, the liberation of inner conflicts. Just learn not to hold back when the journey begins. Go into the experience of feelings and emotions the way you dive into water. Remember not to apply those classical, religious judgments toward emotions as being instinctual, sinful or dirty. Experience whatever arises without judgment, pleasure or pain, lust or depression, love or anger.

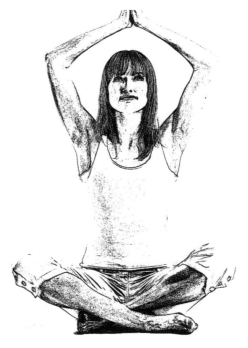

Here are some methods that will allow you to connect with your feelings. After you have done some stretching exercise, like Yoga, shake your body from head to foot. While you are shaking, breathe fast and deep for a while and also make sounds such as "Ha". Sitting in the lotus position, focus on your breathing. When you inhale, imagine that you're entering into you emotions and feelings. Imagine a powerful event in your life which ignited the emotions. Let the feeling develop fully.

Mind is like a wild monkey. It jumps from one place to another place. It repeats the same stuff and now and then it imagines new things too. Mind or consciousness is enigmatic phenomena. We do have power over it and we do not. We could try to direct our thoughts and eventually the thoughts would win. We do not remember how and when we lost concentration. Thoughts can be both comforting and intrusive. When a thought is comforting we have more positive thoughts, like fantasies or positive thoughts about ourselves. Sometimes we have negative imagination and dreadful thoughts. Our mind is like traffic. It is congested with familiar and unfamiliar thoughts.

There was a famous Tibetan lama who used to meditate and count his thoughts the whole day. When he had a positive thought, he would pick up a white stone. When he had a negative thought, he would pick up a black stone. First he got only black stones but gradually all he got were white ones. The black stones represented judgment of the arising thought as being negative. The white stones represented states of non-judgment towards arising thoughts. Remember this story is not about getting rid of bad thoughts, nor keeping good thoughts, rather about becoming aware of the thought process and more and more free of judgment, of liking or disliking thoughts. Eventually one will develop a state when one neither thinks of thoughts as being positive or negative but simply dwells in the pure awareness of thoughts.

Consciousness mindfulness is becoming aware of every process of thought, yet not judging nor attempting to capture particular ones or push other ones away. That is a form of resistance. Thoughts are just thoughts. They are not good or bad. It is a liberating experience to simply let the thoughts arise without controlling them or preferring one over another. Be a witness of the thought process. Be fascinated by the process of your own thoughts just the way you are fascinated by the beauty of the setting sun.

Many meditators try to push away negative thoughts. When one tries to stop thoughts, thoughts become intrusive and neurotic. It is the same as telling someone not to imagine a monkey, but what happens is that one ends up thinking about the monkey. Do not fight your mind with your mind, because it is not a separate entity from you.

Here are a few steps for consciousness mindfulness meditation:-

- After sitting in a comfortable posture, focus on the breath.
- Keep your mind clear and vigilant, do not let yourself feel sleepy or too relaxed which happens during meditation.
- Let all thoughts arise spontaneously, even if they are sometimes disturbing.
- Do not attach or be disturbed by any of them. If you have a thought of saving the whole world or of stealing your neighbour's cute puppy, do not judge them.
- Just laugh when you see all these contradictions of the mind. Then you will be liberated from your own thoughts.

If you want to be free from suffering, you must realise reality, the way that things are. There is no way to find salvation or liberation outside. There is no supernatural being or holy man who can grab your hand and take away all your problems.

Even Buddha says:-

"I can only show the path to liberation, but liberation itself depends on you."

Human suffering is a form of nightmare. It does not really exist, as we perceive it. If you inquire about the nature of suffering, where is it? What is it? You will not find its existence outside of yourself. Suffering, pain and sorrow, all of them exist in your own mind. If you are not free from your own mind, you will never find happiness anywhere by escaping from one circumstance and changing to another.

Buddha says:-

"Mind is the creator of everything"

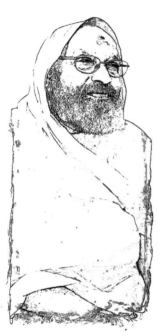

The very cause of happiness and suffering is in one's own mind. You cannot go beyond anything unless you can cut through the cause in your mind. The cause is known as ignorance, the lack of understanding of reality. The duality of happiness and suffering, good and bad is created by our own minds. The duality does not exist outside of one's mind.

Why do we constantly attempt to alter the conditions of life instead of altering our perspective of life? Dharma, in Tibetan Language is called "choo". Choo means modification. Dharma is a way of modifying one's mind. When we modify our perspective towards everything, there is no need to fix any situation outside of oneself. We try to make our life perfect and super by desiring a more perfect lifestyle, career or relationship. Hope and fear are our main sufferings that dominate our everyday life. Until we go beyond hope and fear, we will relentlessly experience turmoil. Desire to control life is the factor of hope. Fear is the fear of not being able to control it.

First, we need to come to the realisation of everything as our mental projection. Then we have to learn how to be conscious of ourselves, especially the way we react to situations based on our own hope and fear.

The idea of phenomena mindfulness is to see the way that things are without distortion, the distortions of our own projections and perceptions. To do that, we have to understand that we are bound by our own delusions and that we react from that point of view. With this awareness we have the perfect means with which to eliminate our conflict and suffering. The moment we are consciously aware of our own delusion, the delusion begins to fade. Under the circumstances we need not try to eradicate our delusion by exerting effort or, so called, spiritual discipline. The very reason we do all sorts of spiritual practice, such as meditation, yoga and different forms of exercise, is to become conscious of our own delusions and neurosis.

Once we become a conscious person we are becoming more an enlightened one, a Buddha. Buddha means awakened one or conscious being, but does not mean one who is completely immaculate and who does not have to go through any process of purification. When we are able to be mindful of everything around us, we are able to see clearly the way things are. We see everything as impermanent and transient. We begin to know that there is no reason to be attached to anything in this world, since everything is disappearing in every moment.

We no longer are attached to our thoughts, emotions, life style and relationships. Nothing exists longer than a moment anyway. Attachment comes into being by obsessing with our memory about the past. Non-attachment is not about being insensitive. It's a state where we can experience love and joy by not being attached to our internal obscurations.

Here are stages for the Meditation:-

- Hold the intention to let go of all of your attachment to your thoughts and emotions whenever you are ready to practice the meditation.

- When you have the thought to meditate, just meditate right at that moment, no matter wherever you are or whatever you're doing, even if you are fighting with someone on the telephone or jumping in the air.

- Focus on the breath and imagine that the belly is the place where you breathe.

- Every time you attach to your thoughts or emotions, breathe deeply and focus on that.

- Mindfulness meditation-the simple step-by-step approach

1. Take a few minutes to stop what you are doing and focus your attention onto the flow of thoughts in your mind. Pay particular attention to thoughts that have an emotional charge, such as an impulse to get angry or to become irritated or frustrated. Most of the time, we find ourselves compelled to react whenever these kind of thought-impulses arise. Somehow, we are convinced that we have to become angry if that drive cuts in front of us, or disappointed if a project fails, or worried about our finances. But the truth of the matter is that there is absolutely no law that says that we have to react that way and suffer accordingly. The reason we suffer is because we have become slaves to our negative thoughts, beliefs and conditioned emotional reactions. They run our lives not through choice but through ignorance and unawareness. We need to regain choice about what we want to feel in our lives.

2. Now, if you respond to your compulsive emotions with kindness and give them lots of space, then they will respond by unclenching, unwinding and becoming malleable like moist clay. Mindfulness is the healing energy that moistens that which is brittle and hard. Many compulsions will heal themselves if you don't proliferate further reactivity. Give

them lots of space and they will dissipate by themselves.

3. Cultivate and sustain this spacious quality of mindfulness with your anger, irritation, disappointment, hurt, anxiety, worry and each of the many stress producing reactions and you effectively neutralise the whole reactive process. If you stop feeding the stress reactions with reactive thinking they will lose their momentum and begin to dissolve away. They become irrelevant and before long you will wonder what all the bother was about. What you are doing is learning to neutralise your habitual reactivity by cultivating awareness of each reaction, and in this simple awareness you create space in which emotions can defuse themselves and resolve.

4. Stress is the product of negative habitual reactions to life events, and as you blindly repeat these learned reaction they become habitual. You need to begin repeating the positive responses you experience through mindfulness training.   Repeat these more positive responses as often as possible, and try to establish new habits that defuse stress and allow more creative thinking and problem-solving. The mindfulness response grows quickly through repetition, and every time you touch suffering with mindfulness you strengthen the path towards inner freedom from suffering and stress. When you are stuck with the process or feeling that you are not getting the benefit you should be getting, go back to step 1.

5. The moment you get the sense of mindfulness, carry that throughout your entire day with worldly and spiritual activities.

For mindfulness meditation to work effectively it requires a fair degree of time and practice. By far the best option is to join a group that uses mindfulness meditation so that you can learn from them and join them in learning and practising all of the steps involved. If you choose to join a group, it is almost certain you will derive a great deal of benefit both from being able to share in the group's knowledge of the subject itself, as well as being able to discuss it and socialise with like-minded people.

TASKS

At the end of Chapter 9 we have outlined some simple steps for you to take to begin mindfulness meditation, without having to go through the more time consuming and exhaustive process of learning this technique in a more comprehensive fashion.

Go through these simple steps, and immediately afterwards fill in a Mood Compass. We trust and hope that when you compare this Mood compass with previous ones you will be able to see the considerable improvement in the balance of the bodily and emotional feelings.

CHAPTER TEN

EMOTIONAL FREEDOM TECHNIQUES

"We expected the acupuncture to improve the pain. We didn't really expect the largest benefit to be in fatigue or anxiety."

David Martin

Emotional Freedom technique is a relatively new therapy that has been applied in many cases of Bipolar Disorder. EFT is sometimes known as tapping, or even energy tapping. People describe this therapy as a form of energy psychology using acupuncture principles to balance the body's energy system. This is done by tapping on the body's acupressure points, sometimes with a EFT specialist but it can also be done by oneself after suitable training.

There have been mixed successes with EFT, perhaps unsurprising in view of the newness of this technique and the fact that it is still developing. EFT certainly does work very well in cases of anxiety, phobias and general negative thought patterns. It has also been shown to have a very positive effect on depression and can certainly live mood very effectively when applied properly. Experience has shown that EFT is also very helpful in cases of chronic pain. Bipolar Disorder is not quite so straightforward, in that it is of course a disorder of opposites, both depression and mania. Therapists generally suggest that when a manic episode is in progress EFT is unlikely to be able to halt it. However, regular use of the technique is likely to prevent the manic episode from occurring in the first place. Even if an episode is felt to be coming on, the early use of EFT techniques can prevent it from developing into a full-blown mania. This also applies in the case of depression, where when the episode is at its most severe EFT is not likely to be totally ineffective. However before the episode of depression begins, or when it is detected in its very early stages, EFT can often either prevent the episode from occurring at all or mitigate the very worst of its symptoms.

You should therefore regard EFT as one very valuable tool in your collection of tools and techniques to deal with your disorder. There is absolutely no doubt that you will derive greater benefit from applying this therapy, whilst at the same time accepting an understanding that it is not in itself a complete solution. Before we look into the actual techniques of applying EFT, let us examine the little advantages of this therapy.

- EFT can rapidly eliminate emotional turmoil before it spirals out of control.
- EFT can reduce or eliminate feelings of anger and rage.
- EFT can eliminate feelings of helplessness, hopelessness and powerlessness, together with feelings of guilt and shame.
- EFT is very effective in reducing or even eliminating the side effect of anxiety that often presents itself during a Bipolar attack.

- EFT can help to sort out past emotional difficulties, the kind that can trigger further emotional difficulties that lead to Bipolar attack.
- EFT can in turn help you to become aware of these old emotional difficulties, to get rid of them and avoid them recurring in the future.
- EFT is empowering, it will help you to take control and stop being a victim.
- EFT can help you to alter negative and distorted thoughts, and re-establish positive and more helpful thought patterns.
- EFT will help you to achieve a calmness and peace.

As you can see, EFT offers a huge range of benefits and advantages, so much so that you should regard it as an essential part of your therapy for Bipolar Disorder. The therapy was originally rooted in ancient Chinese medicine. The Chinese believed that we have an energy body with energy flowing through it along lines called meridians. When these meridians became blocked the result was the body became ill. The Chinese identified a great number of different points on his physical body that could be stimulated sufficiently to influence health. There are several other therapies both ancient and new that are related to this meridians theory, including acupuncture, acupressure, reflexology and a range of other energy therapies. By comparison to almost any other process, EFT is quite gentle and rarely has any side effects. It is often used instead of other procedures, because of its gentle nature.

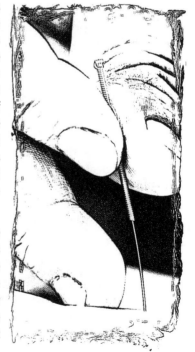

The development of "emotional acupuncture", as it is sometimes referred to, was indirectly assisted by Dr George Goodheart, a well known chiropractor in the United States who founded a branch of chiropractic based upon a precise method of testing the body for information about its own needs. Goodheart had learned about acupuncture in 1962 from reading an interesting book written by the president of the Acupuncture Society in Britain. He was intrigued with the possibilities it promised for his own practice. He then studied acupuncture and soon introduced it into his own work as one of the bases of a new method he was developing called Applied Kinesiology (which uses muscle testing to determine the appropriateness of any form of treatment).

Substituting simple manual pressure for needles, he found that he could obtain the same beneficial results by simply applying manual pressure to the acupuncture points, or by "percussing" or "tapping" on them. This advance made the acupuncture-derived method accessible to many more people, since it was non-invasive. Building on the work of Goodheart, in the 1970's an Australian psychiatrist

John Diamond MD took this discovery a step further. He created a variation of it which he called "Behavioral Kinesiology". This derivative of Goodheart's method added an interesting component. Diamond used affirmations, positive self-statements or thoughts, when the person was contacting selected acupuncture points, and did this specifically to treat emotional problems. His innovative departure in this respect foreshadowed the later development of the "meridian-based therapies" and Energy Psychology, in the forefront of which we find EFT today.

But before EFT could be invented, another step was necessary. The concept of using tapping of acupoints to treat psychological problems needed a structure to become widely applicable. This structure was supplied by an American psychologist, Dr Roger Callahan, who specialised in anxiety disorders. In the early 1980's Dr Callahan learned Applied Kinesiology and studied the meridian system of acupuncture in an effort to find better answers to some of the problems his patients faced, particularly those of anxiety and phobias. He then took the step that was necessary to bring the tapping procedures into a full fledged form of psychological treatment, by combining the use of "tapping" for emotional problems with simultaneous focusing on the problem at hand. Callahan had discovered that if a person is focusing on a specific fear of their own at the time they tap this fear can be removed, often permanently.

Dr Callahan's new treatment came into being after he studied the meridian system, but it was an unexpected occurrence which led to the precise clinical discovery that foreshadowed the later development of EFT.

Callahan had been working for over two years with Mary, a patient of his who had such an overwhelming fear of water that she could not even get into a bathtub without this precipitating an anxiety attack. Although he had tried many anxiety reduction techniques with her, the progress had been slow and discouraging. Mary could not even approach the swimming pool in the grounds of his office or allow water to contact her body, without experiencing panic.

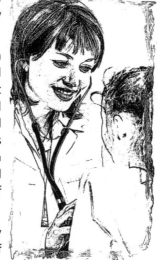

One day however, while they were working on this fear in his office, Mary told him for the first time that she felt the fearful in her stomach. As it happens, there is an acupuncture point located directly beneath the eye which, according to traditional acupuncture, is linked to the stomach meridian. Dr Callahan asked her to tap on that point. He did this on the assumption that this manoeuver might balance a possible disturbance in her meridian energy system and thereby lessen her stomach symptoms. He had no idea that it would have profound implications for the future of his practice and for psychology.

Mary agreed to tap under her eyes and when she did so a totally unexpected thing happened. Instead of merely experiencing relief from her stomach symptoms, she called out in surprise that her fear of water had suddenly gone! Callahan did not take this too seriously at first because it seemed so unlikely, but then he watched her get up and run toward the swimming pool. When she reached it, she began splashing water on her face, he then took notice. She had never been able to go near the pool before.

It is common to use affirmations during the process of EFT, or tapping, to link the power of EFT to the emotions. The combination of tapping the energy meridians and voicing positive affirmation works to clear the short circuit, the emotional block, from your body's bio-energy system, thus restoring your mind and body's balance. This is essential for optimal health and the healing of physical disease.

Some people are initially wary of these principles that EFT is based on. This being electromagnetic energy that flows through the body and regulates our health. It is only recently becoming recognized. Others are initially taken aback by, and sometimes amused by, the EFT tapping and affirmation methodology, whose basics you will learn here. However, it is because of its very high rate of success that the use of EFT has spread rapidly. Medical practitioners using it are now found worldwide.

The basic EFT sequence is straightforward and generally takes patients only a few minutes to learn. While it is important to tap the correct area, you need not worry about being absolutely precise, as tapping the general area is sufficient.

The first thing to understand is that you will be tapping with your fingers. There are a number of acupuncture meridians on your fingertips. When you tap with your fingertips you are also likely using not only the meridians you are tapping on, but also the ones on your fingers.

Traditional EFT has you tapping with the fingertips of your index finger and middle finger and with only one hand. Either hand works just as well. Most of the tapping points exist on either side of the body. It does not matter which side you use, nor does it matter if you switch sides during the tapping. For example, you can tap under your right eye and, later in the tapping, under your left arm.

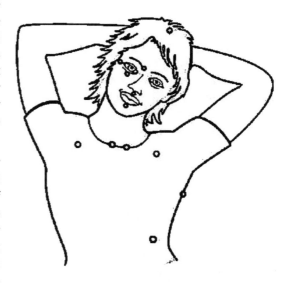

You can use both hands and all your fingers, so that they are gently relaxed and form a slightly curved natural line. The use of more fingers allows you to access more of the acupuncture points. When you use all your fingers you will cover a larger area than just tapping with one or two fingertips. This will allow you to cover the tapping points more easily. However, many obtain quite successful results with the traditional one-handed two-finger approach. Either method can be used.

Use your fingertips, not your finger pads, as they have more meridian points. However, if you have long fingernails you should of course use your finger pads (otherwise you may end up stabbing yourself). You should also remove your watch and bracelets, as that will interfere with your use of the wrist meridian tapping.

You should tap solidly, but never so hard as to hurt or bruise yourself. If you decide to use both hands, slightly alternating the tapping so that each hand is slightly out of phase with the other and you are not tapping with both hands simultaneously. This provides a kinesthetic variant of the alternating eye movement work that is done in EMDR and may have some slight additional benefit.

When you tap on the points outlined below, you will tap about 5-7 times. The actual number is not critical, but ideally should be about the length of time it takes for one full breath. There is probably a distinct benefit for tapping through one complete respiration cycle.

These tapping points proceed down the body. Each tapping point is below the one before it, which should make it easier to remember. However, unlike TFT, the sequence is not critical. You can tap the points in any order and sequence, just so long as all the points are covered. It just is easier to go from top to bottom to make sure you remember to do them all.

Glasses and watches can mechanically and electromagnetically interfere with EFT, so remove them prior to tapping. For quick sessions on yourself this is not so critical.

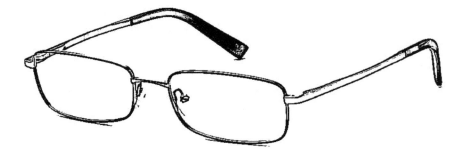

Many people are concerned about embarrassing themselves by using EFT in public. After a while of using and perfecting the technique, in private if you prefer, you will be able to use only two fingers of one hand and to say the affirmation softly under your breath or even silently. This way you can do EFT in just about any social setting, and if people even notice what you are doing at all, it will appear to them that you are merely thinking.

The tapping points, and their abbreviations, are explained below, followed by a chart of the points. They are presented below in the exact order in which they should be tapped.

1. Top of the Head (TH)

With fingers back to back down the centre of the skull.

2. Eyebrow (EB)

Just above and to one side of the nose, at the beginning of the eyebrow.

3. Side of the Eye (SE)

On the bone bordering the outside corner of the eye.

4. Under the Eye (UE)

On the bone under an eye about one inch below your pupil.

5. Under the Nose (UN)

On the small area between the bottom of your nose and the top of your upper lip.

6. Chin (Ch)

Midway between the point of your chin and the bottom of your lower lip. Even though it is not directly on the point of the chin, it is called the chin point because it is easier to understand.

7. Collar Bone (CB)

The junction where the sternum (breastbone), collarbone and the first rib meet. This is a very important point and in acupuncture is referred to as K (kidney) 27. To locate it, first place your forefinger on the U-shaped notch at the top of the breastbone (about where a man would knot his tie). From the bottom of the U, move your forefinger down toward the navel one inch and then go to the left (or right) one inch. This point is referred to as Collar Bone even though it is not on the collarbone (or clavicle) per se.

8. Under the Arm (UA)

On the side of the body, at a point even with the nipple (for men) or in the middle of the bra strap (for women). It is about four inches below the armpit.

9. Wrists (WR)

The last point is the inside of both wrists.

- TH Top of Head
- EB Eye Brow
- SE Side of the Eye
- UE Under the Eye
- UN Under the Nose
- Ch Chin

- CB   Collar Bone
- UA   Under the Arm
- WR Wrists

Now that you understand how to actually perform the mechanical tapping and where you need to tap, you will next need to know what to say while you are tapping.

The traditional EFT phrase uses the following setup:-

"Even though I have this _____,

I deeply and completely accept myself."

You can also substitute this as the second part of the phrase:

"I deeply and completely love and accept myself."

Fill on the blank with a brief description of the addiction, food craving, negative emotion or other problem you want to address.

Examples Using the Traditional EFT Phrasing

While these examples represent a range of problems, keep in mind there really is no limit to the types of issues you can confront with EFT:-

- "Even though I have this fear of public speaking, I deeply and completely accept myself."
- "Even though I have this headache, I deeply and completely accept myself."
- "Even though I have this anger towards my father, I deeply and completely accept myself."
- "Even though I have this war memory, I deeply and completely accept myself."
- "Even though I have this stiffness in my neck, I deeply and completely accept myself."
- "Even though I have these nightmares, I deeply and completely accept myself."
- "Even though I have this craving for alcohol, I deeply and completely accept myself."
- "Even though I have this fear of snakes, I deeply and completely accept myself."
- "Even though I have this depression, I deeply and completely accept myself."

OTHER EFT PHRASE OPTIONS

You can also try these other phrase variations. All of these affirmations are correct because they follow the same general format. They acknowledge the problem and create self-acceptance despite the existence of the problem. That is necessary for the affirmation to be effective.

You can use any of them but the previous ones above are easy to remember and have a good track record at getting the job done.

- "I accept myself even though I have this_____."
- "Even though I have this _____, I deeply and profoundly accept myself."
- "I love and accept myself even though I have this_____."

It does not matter whether you believe the affirmation or not...just say it. It is better to say it with feeling and emphasis, but saying it routinely will usually do the job. It is best to say it out loud, but if you are in a social situation where you prefer to mutter it under your breath...or do it silently...that is fine. It will still likely be effective. To add to the effectiveness of the affirmation, the setup also includes the simultaneous tapping on one of the acupuncture meridian points.

Tuning in is seemingly a very simple process. You merely think about the problem while applying the tapping. That is it, at least in theory. The cause of all negative emotions is a disruption in the body's energy system. Negative emotions come because you are tuned in to certain thoughts or circumstances, which in turn, cause your energy system to disrupt. Otherwise, you function normally. One's fear of heights is not present for example, while reading the comic section of the Sunday newspaper, and therefore not tuned in to the problem. Tuning in to a problem can be done by simply thinking about it. In fact, tuning in means thinking about it. Thinking about the problem will bring about the energy disruptions involved. Without tuning in to the problem, thereby creating those energy disruptions, EFT does nothing.

Now you will need to tap on each of the points described above while you are stating the positive affirmation. This will only take a few moments to do.

You should:-

- Select an appropriate affirmation.
- Carefully "tune in" to your problem by actually trying to hold the problem in your thought.
- State the affirmations in a loud voice with great passion, energy and enthusiasm.

If you do this while tapping the points described earlier, it is highly likely you will notice a major decrease in the issue or problem that you were tapping on. If your problem or issue resolves completely, you are done with the tapping. If it does not decrease or decreases to a level that is less than acceptable, move on to the next section.

Sometimes one round of the tapping sequence, while voicing your affirmation, is enough to clear up the issue. However when subsequent rounds are necessary, you can employ a reminder phrase. This is simply a word or short phrase that describes the problem and which you repeat out loud each time you tap one of the points in the sequence. In this way you continually remind your system about the problem you are working on.

The best reminder phrase to use is usually identical to what you choose for the affirmation you initially used. However you can use a short cut, if the setup is particularly long, by simply saying one or several words to speed up the process and do more rounds.

For example if you are working on a fear of public speaking, the initial or setup affirmation would go like this:-

"Even though I have this fear of public speaking,
I deeply and completely accept myself."

Within this affirmation, the underlined words "fear of public speaking" are ideal for use as the reminder phrase. Simply repeating this reminder phrase and the affirmation are usually sufficient to tune into the problem at hand.

Sometimes the first round of tapping does not completely eliminate a problem. This may be because a new issue or issues that prevent further progress show themselves via the tapping. These issues, whether images, conversations, interactions or in some other form, are in some way related to the first problem being addressed. Sometimes they are part of or the core of the cause, sometimes they are a result. The barrier restricting your emotional health, in other words, is made up of more than one brick and you must eliminate all the bricks.

If this is the case, you should do additional rounds of tapping as necessary to eliminate all the issues, but adjust your affirmation slightly as follows for best results:-

> *"Even though I still have some of this _____,*
> *I deeply and completely accept myself."*

Note the words "still" and "some" and how they change the thrust of the affirmation toward the remainder of the problem.

Water conducts electricity and EFT accesses the electrical energy that flows through our bodies and minds. It is very important for you to be properly hydrated. Doing affirmations is one of the best ways to be kind to your mind. Every thought you have, every sentence you speak is an affirmation of a sort. It is either positive or negative. However, you can also do specific intentional affirmations. And the god thing about doing affirmations is that you can radically improve the effectiveness with EFT.

You can do this by first creating a definite positive statement that builds you up. We are talking about definite positive statements to make or do, something in our lives or to create a specific goal. You can start this process with positive self-statements. Even if it does not feel true to begin with, you will want to do these statements or affirmations many times a day. When you wake up, when you go to bed, every time you go to the bathroom you should say them. It is especially important to tap and say the affirmations before you go to sleep. This is probably the single most important time to do it. When you tap before you go to bed you will give your subconscious six to eight hours to work on your affirmations and help create them for you. If you find prayer a helpful resource, you can integrate your prayer into the

EFT SEQUENCES

This is quite simple and inexpensive. All you will need is a mirror and some time. You can tap alone or in the dark. It may be more effective to tap while staring at your own eyes in the mirror. This seems to provide a far deeper connection with your subconscious. It is almost as if the mirror is reflecting your energy back into you rather than going out into space somewhere. If you have not tried this yet you really need to consider using this simple yet powerful technique.

You can begin by looking in the mirror and doing your EFT affirmations and tap on all the EFT points. Pay careful attention and listen to what you hear, especially focusing on any negative messages that can be blocking your progress. Listen and follow through.   Learn to trust yourself.

We frequently have a tendency to be negative about every little thing, no matter how small. We can all use forgiveness on a daily basis and you can use the mirror to help you in this way too. Start by looking into your eyes and say:-

> *"Even though I wasn't successful or I was angry or impatient or mean or cruel….. "*

Or whatever problem you need to forgive yourself for then say:-

- I forgive you, I was only doing the best I could
- I forgive you for holding onto those patterns for to long
- I forgive you for not loving yourself

When you say "you" you are looking directly into your own eyes.

You must try this as it is quite powerful. Remember to always acknowledge the negative thought if it is there, but do not give it a lot of importance. You will then you will want to use EFT on the negative thought that comes up and create a positive opposite. When you first say an affirmation it may not seem to be true. Remember that affirmations are like planting seeds in the ground. It helps if you think of your mind as a garden in which you are planting your thoughts are seeds.

When you make these affirmations think of them as planting new seeds. When you plant a seed in the ground it is only a tiny seed, you do not have a fully grown plant. That little seed needs to germinate. Then it breaks open its little shell and it starts to get nourishment from the earth. Then first the roots come out and then, and only then, does that first little shoot appear. Just like it takes some time for the seed to grow into a plant, it takes some time from your first affirmation to the realisation of your goal. It does not matter whether you see the results or you do not see them. You have to trust that it just takes time.

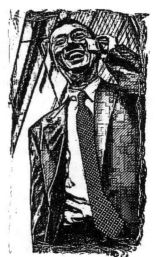

When a fear thought comes, simply say:-

> *"Thanks for sharing, thank you for protecting me."*

Do not give it power. Do not run from it. Whatever comes up, it is very important to acknowledge it, when you hear them you can even write them down. Once you have written the fear though down, you can turn it around to a positive affirmation and tap it in with EFT. You can say:-

> *"Even though I have this fear (name the fear) I deeply love and accept myself and I fully appreciate that it is only trying to help me."*

Then do an affirmation for what you really want, which is typically the positive present tense opposite of the fear, or whatever positive outcome you would desire instead of the fear. Avoid denying the fear. You must always acknowledge the fear. That is the real beauty of EFT. It always acknowledges the truth and helps remove you from the denial trap that so many of us fall into. EFT helps you understand that your fear thought is there to protect you. Fear is there to protect us. It is important to recognise that no matter where you are in life, no matter what you contributed to creating, no matter what is happening, you are always doing the best you can with the understanding, awareness, and knowledge that you have until you can find a better way to handle the situation. A critical truth that is helpful to remember when doing this work is that your persistent and consistent thoughts will eventually become your reality. Focus on positive thoughts

Unfortunately many people do EFT affirmations for a few days, say it does not work and give up. Everything happens in a perfect time space sequence. Trust that. EFT seems to rapidly accelerate not only the time at which your goal is realised, but the likelihood for your success.

Always remember to say your positive statements in the present tense. Your subconscious mind is very literal and if you ask it to do something in the future, you may fail to achieve your for many long years. Many people commonly default to this by force of habit. It takes a conscious effort to avoid this non-intentional self-defeating habit. Always avoid saying you will have or going to have, which is in the future tense. Always say your affirmation in the present tense, otherwise you run the serious risk delay achieving what you want and you may never succeed in this.

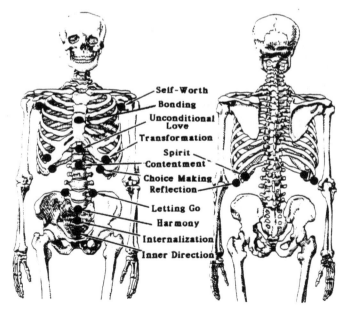

Here is a very heartening letter that was posted recently in an online forum. EFT does work, it works well, and here is strong evidence.

Following is a letter from Lizzie, who came to me with her eight year old daughter Grace. Grace is Romanian. She was adopted when she was two years old. Lizzie wanted me to write about her daughter because there is a good chance that there are many more cases of adopted Romanian girls out there that have problems with anger as they get older.

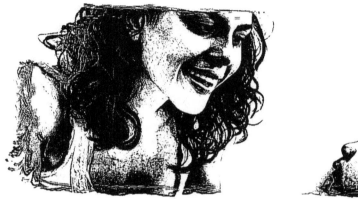
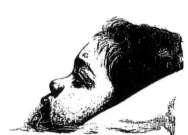

Grace would have severe rage tantrums, where she would hit and kick her parents, especially her mother. She would scream continuously and hit anyone near her. Nothing would calm her down or stop her screaming until she was exhausted. It was very painful, emotionally and physically especially for her mother. It would happen more than once a week and Grace would totally out of control. She had no friends, other children and their parents were afraid of her.

"My daughter grace is nine years old. She has had five years of therapy (three different ones). She has been diagnosed as Bipolar Disease and a Re-active Disorder. She has extremely violent episodes several times a week. She is treated by a child psychiatrist and is heavily medicated. At our wits end we decided to try EFT. We have had two sessions and are already seeing more improvement than with all the other therapies combined.

We still have a long way to go, but for the first time in many years we have hope that our daughter can have a normal life."

When Grace and her mother came into my office we all started tapping on the sternum. We all kept doing this throughout the visit.

When asked what she felt when she was really angry Grace said she felt tight and hungry. This made sense as she had been found on the street as toddler and was taken to an orphanage, where she stayed until she was adopted.

184

I asked her to lift her arms and shout with me again and again "I am very angry" until I noticed subtle changes in her face. We then changed to "I am angry and I'm very hungry" and she started crying. Her mother was amazed as she had never seen her cry before. She was unaware Grace felt hungry when angry. We decided that from now on Amanda would always have some snack in her pocket in case she ever got hungry or angry when not at home. Grace liked that idea, nodded repeatedly and even had a small smile.

This was in the first 15 minutes of our first session.

Grace then drew me a picture of what angry and happy looks like to her. By then she was happy to follow instructions. We agreed that she and her mother would do a few rounds of tapping every night at bedtime.

We ended the first session tapping on:-

- Even though I am very hungry, I'm cool.
- Even though I am hungry when I'm angry, I promise to eat my snacks because I'm a very cool kid.
- Eating makes me feel good and I won't have to scream and hit my mum.
- Even though I feel very angry sometimes and I scare the other kids in school, from now on I will eat when I'm hungry. Eating calms me down and makes me feel much better because I don't want the others to be scared of me. I want them to be my friends.
- I love my mum and I don't want to hurt her because she loves me very much.

During the week between sessions she had another anger episode, but this time no hitting or kicking. She just screamed for a whole hour. This was bad enough for her parents. The reasons for her screaming are always little things, if she is told she can't do or have something, or a change of routine. Grace cannot cope with changes easily. The anger tantrums are a cry for help and there is enormous pressure behind them. Before she came to see me she would not let her mother hold her or touch her in any way during her rages. I now have her mother tap herself, Grace is still unable to be touched during her screaming fits. The latest fit was very much shorter, no hitting or kicking, and Lizzie made her to laugh and stop while she tapped right in front of her. That was enormous progress.

We established a new rule that Grace has to into the garden if she feels anger coming on. She will shout out there something like "I am so angry, but I am going to tap now..... I soon will calm down. This little girl will only accept what makes sense to her. This is huge a challenge for her parents every day. She is highly intelligent and comes from a very different culture. This needs to be considered in order to understand and connect with her. I am very confident that she will eventually make a full recovery from this dreadful time and enjoy her homelife with her loving parents and to fully intergrate at school and socially. Some day the medical profession will wake up and realize that unresolved emotional issues are the main cause of 85% of all illnesses. When they do, EFT will be one of their primary healing tools - as it is for me." Eric Robins, MD

Emotional Freedom Techniques are clearly not a simple shortcut to relief from the worst of your Bipolar symptoms. However, at the end of Chapter 10 we hope that we have convinced you of the value of EFT.

TASKS

Your task at the end of this chapter is to find a group that uses EFT therapy and explore the possibilities of joining the group and benefiting from the expertise that they have to offer. You should also fill in a final Mood Compass and keep this with the previous ones.

If you have managed to locate a suitable source of EFT therapy, it would be extremely valuable to fill in a further Mood Compass after you have been for your first session and compare it with the last one you filled in before you went for that session to gain an overview of how useful the therapy was for you. If there is no group to you to join and you need to find a therapist, you should be able to find one who is offering the first session free so that you can try it this therapy without any kind of expense or commitment.

Now that you have completed all of the chapters and steps in this book, you should be well on the way towards a massive relief from the symptoms you are suffering from Bipolar Disorder. Depending on the severity of your disorder and your physical and emotional makeup, it may well be that you have overcome the symptoms completely. At the other end of the spectrum, if your symptoms are more severe and difficult to cope with, at the very least you will have gained a hugely valuable set of tools and techniques that will help you to anticipate future attacks of depression and mania and reduce their severity.

We wish you the very best of good health. You should be proud that you have taken such a strong step to overcome your disorder when so many others are less proactive and more likely to continue suffering for mich of their lives.

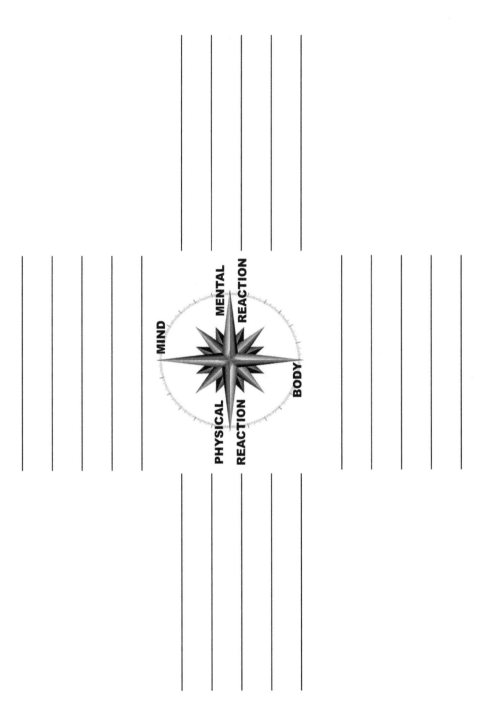

GLOSSARY

Abnormal: Not normal. Deviating from the usual structure, position, condition, or behavior. In referring to a growth, abnormal may mean that it is cancerous or premalignant (likely to become cancer).

Acquired: Anything that is not present at birth but develops some time later. In medicine, the word "acquired" implies "new" or "added." An acquired condition is "new" in the sense that it is not genetic (inherited) and "added" in the sense that was not present at birth.

Acquired immunodeficiency syndrome: AIDS. AIDS is a disease due to infection with the human immunodeficiency virus (HIV). Also referred to as acquired immunodeficiency disease.

Acute: Of abrupt onset, in reference to a disease. Acute often also connotes an illness that is of short duration, rapidly progressive, and in need of urgent care.

ADHD: Attention deficit hyperactivity disorder .

American Psychiatric Association: A medical specialty society with over 35,000 US and international member physicians who "work together to ensure humane care and effective treatment for all persons with mental disorder, including mental retardation and substance-related disorders. It is the voice and conscience of modern psychiatry. Its vision is a society that has available, accessible quality psychiatric diagnosis and treatment." The American Psychiatric Association (APA) is the oldest national medical specialty society in the US.

Anorexia: An eating disorder characterized by markedly reduced appetite or total aversion to food. Anorexia is a serious psychological disorder. It is a condition that goes well beyond out-of-control dieting. The person with anorexia, most often a girl or young woman, initially begins dieting to lose weight. Over time, the weight loss becomes a sign of mastery and control. The drive to become thinner is thought to be secondary to concerns about control and fears relating to one's body. The individual continues the endless cycle of restrictive eating, often to a point close to starvation. This becomes an obsession and is similar to an addiction to a drug. Anorexia can be life-threatening. Also called anorexia nervosa .

Anorexia nervosa: See Anorexia .

Antidepressant: Anything, and especially a drug, used to prevent or treat depression.

Antihypertensive: Something that reduces high blood pressure (hypertension).

Antipsychotic: A medication (or another measure) that is believed to be effective in the treatment of psychosis . For example, aripiprazole (Abilify) is an antipsychotic medication used to treat schizophrenia .

Anxiety: A feeling of apprehension and fear characterized by physical symptoms such as palpitations , sweating, and feelings of stress . Anxiety disorders are serious medical illnesses that affect approximately 19 million American adults. These disorders fill people's lives with overwhelming anxiety and fear. Unlike the relatively mild, brief anxiety caused by a stressful event such as a business presentation or a first date, anxiety disorders are chronic, relentless, and can grow progressively worse if not treated.

Atypical: Not typical, not usual, not normal, abnormal. Atypical is often used to refer to the appearance of precancerous or cancerous cells.

Bipolar disorder : A mood disorder sometimes called manic-depressive illness or manic-depression that characteristically involves cycles of depression and elation or mania . Sometimes the mood switches from high to low and back again are dramatic and rapid, but more often they are gradual and slow, and intervals of normal mood may occur between the high (manic) and low (depressive) phases of the condition. The symptoms of both the depressive and manic cycles may be severe and often lead to impaired functioning.

Birth control : Birth control is the use of any practices, methods, or devices to prevent pregnancy from occurring in a sexually active woman. Also referred to as family planning, pregnancy prevention, fertility control, or contraception; birth control methods are designed either to prevent fertilization of an egg or implantation of a fertilized egg in the uterus.

Blood clot: Blood that has been converted from a liquid to a solid state. Also called a thrombus .

Blood clots: Blood that has been converted from a liquid to a solid state. Also called a thrombus.

Blood count: The calculated number of white or red blood cells (WBCs or RBCs) in a cubic millimeter of blood.

Blood sugar: Blood glucose . See also: High blood sugar ; Low blood sugar .

Brain: That part of the central nervous system that is located within the cranium (skull). The brain functions as the primary receiver, organizer and distributor of information for the body. It has two (right and left) halves called "hemispheres."

Brain tumor : A benign or malignant growth in the brain. Primary brain tumors arise in brain tissue. Secondary brain tumors are cancers that have spread to the brain tissue (metastasized) from elsewhere in the body. Brain tumors can and do occur at any age.

Breastfeeding: Feeding a child human breast milk . According to the American Academy of Pediatrics , human breast milk is preferred for all infants. This includes even premature and sick babies, with rare exceptions. It is the food least likely to cause allergic reactions; it is inexpensive; it is readily available at any hour of the day or night; babies accept the taste readily; and the antibodies in breast milk can help a baby resist infections.

Bulimia: Also called bulimia nervosa. An eating disorder characterized by episodes of secretive excessive eating (binge-eating) followed by inappropriate methods of weight control, such as self-induced vomiting (purging), abuse of laxatives and diuretics, or excessive exercise. The insatiable appetite of bulimia is often interrupted by periods of anorexia.

Capsule: Capsule has many meanings in medicine including the following:

1.   In medicine, a membranous structure that envelops an organ, a joint, tumor, or any other part of the body. It is usually made up of dense collagen-containing connective tissue.
2.   In pharmacy, a solid dosage form in which the drug is enclosed in a hard or soft soluble container, usually of a form of gelatin.
3.   In microbiology, a coat around a microbe, such as a bacterium or fungus.

Cell: The basic structural and functional unit in people and all living things. Each cell is a small container of chemicals and water wrapped in a membrane .

Chronic: This important term in medicine comes from the Greek chronos, time and means lasting a long time.

Chronic pain : Pain (an unpleasant sense of discomfort) that persists or progresses over a long period of time. In contrast to acute pain that arises suddenly in response to a specific injury and is usually treatable, chronic pain persists over time and is often resistant to medical treatments.

Cocaine: The most potent stimulant of natural origin, a bitter addictive anesthetic (pain blocker) which is extracted from the leaves of the coca scrub (Erythroxylon coca) indigenous to the Andean highlands of South America.

Constipation: Infrequent (and frequently incomplete) bowel movements. The opposite of diarrhea, constipation is commonly caused by irritable bowel syndrome, diverticulosis, and medications (constipation can paradoxically be caused by overuse of laxatives). Colon cancer can narrow the colon and thereby cause constipation. The large bowel (colon) can be visualized by barium enema x-rays, sigmoidoscopy, and colonoscopy. Barring a condition such as cancer, high-fiber diets can frequently relieve the constipation.

CT scan: Computerized tomography scan. Pictures of structures within the body created by a computer that takes the data from multiple X-ray images and turns them into pictures on a screen. CT stands for computerized tomography.

Cure:

4. 1. To heal, to make well, to restore to good health. Cures are easy to claim and, all too often, difficult to confirm.
5. 2. A time without recurrence of a disease so that the risk of recurrence is small, as in the 5-year cure rate for malignant melanoma.
6. 3. Particularly in the past, a course of treatment. For example, take a cure at a spa.

Dehydration : Excessive loss of body water. Diseases of the gastrointestinal tract that cause vomiting or diarrhea may, for example, lead to dehydration. There are a number of other causes of dehydration including heat exposure, prolonged vigorous exercise (e.g., in a marathon), kidney disease, and medications (diuretics).

Depression : An illness that involves the body, mood, and thoughts, that affects the way a person eats and sleeps, the way one feels about oneself, and the way one thinks about things. A depressive disorder is not the same as a passing blue mood. It is not a sign of personal weakness or a condition that can be wished away. People with a depressive disease cannot merely "pull themselves together" and get better. Without treatment, symptoms can last for weeks, months, or years. Appropriate treatment, however, can help most people with depression.

Diabetes: Refers to diabetes mellitus or, less often, to diabetes insipidus . Diabetes mellitus and diabetes insipidus share the name "diabetes" because they are both conditions characterized by excessive urination (polyuria).

Diagnosis: 1 The nature of a disease ; the identification of an illness. 2 A conclusion or decision reached by diagnosis. The diagnosis is rabies . 3 The identification of any problem. The diagnosis was a plugged IV.

Diarrhea : A familiar phenomenon with unusually frequent or unusually liquid bowel movements, excessive watery evacuations of fecal material. The opposite of constipation . The word "diarrhea" with its odd spelling is a near steal from the Greek "diarrhoia" meaning "a flowing through." Plato and Aristotle may have had diarrhoia while today we have diarrhea. There are myriad infectious and noninfectious causes of diarrhea.

Dizziness: Painless head discomfort with many possible causes including disturbances of vision, the brain, balance (vestibular) system of the inner ear, and gastrointestinal system. Dizziness is a medically indistinct term which laypersons use to describe a variety of conditions ranging from lightheadedness, unsteadiness to vertigo .

Dopamine: An important neurotransmitter (messenger) in the brain.

Dry mouth: The condition of not having enough saliva to keep the mouth wet. This is due to inadequate function of the salivary glands. Everyone has dry mouth once in a while when they are nervous, upset or under stress. But if someone has a dry mouth most all of the time, it can be uncomfortable and lead to serious health problems.

Dysfunction: Difficult function or abnormal function.

EEG: Electroencephalogram, e technique for studying the electrical current within the brain. Electrodes are attached to the scalp. Wires attach these electrodes to a machine which records the electrical impulses. The results are either printed out or displayed on a computer screen. Electroencephalogram is abbreviated EEG.

Electroencephalogram: A study of electrical current within the brain. Electrodes are attached to the scalp. Wires attach these electrodes to a machine which records the electrical impulses. The results are either printed out or displayed on a computer screen. Electroencephalogram is abbreviated EEG.

Emergency department: The department of a hospital responsible for the provision of medical and surgical care to patients arriving at the hospital in need of immediate care. Emergency department personnel may also respond to certain situations within the hospital such cardiac arrests.

Encephalitis: Inflammation of the brain. Encephalitis occurs, for example, in 1 in 1,000 cases of measles . It may start (up to 3 weeks) after onset of the measles rash and present with high fever , convulsions, and coma. It usually runs a blessedly short course with full recovery within a week. Or it may eventuate in central nervous system impairment or death.

Epilepsy (seizure disorder): When nerve cells in the brain fire electrical impulses at a rate of up to four times higher than normal, this causes a sort of electrical storm in the brain, known as a seizure. A pattern of repeated seizures is referred to as epilepsy . Known causes include head injuries, brain tumors, lead poisoning, maldevelopment of the brain, genetic and infectious illnesses. But in fully half of cases, no cause can be found. Medication controls seizures for the majority of patients.

Euphoria: Elevated mood. Euphoria is a desirable and natural occurrence when it results from happy or exciting events. An excessive degree of euphoria that is not linked to events is characteristic of hypomania or mania, abnormal mood states associated with bipolar disorders.

Extrapyramidal side effects: Physical symptoms, including tremor , slurred speech, akathisia, dystonia , anxiety, distress, paranoia, and bradyphrenia, that are primarily associated with improper dosing of or unusual reactions to neuroleptic (anti-psychotic) medications.

Fever : Although a fever technically is any body temperature above the normal of 98.6 degrees F. (37 degrees C.), in practice a person is usually not considered to have a significant fever until the temperature is above 100.4 degrees F (38 degrees C.).

Gene: The basic biological unit of heredity . A segment of deoxyribonucleic acid (DNA) needed to contribute to a function.

Genetic: Having to do with genes and genetic information.

Grief: The normal process of reacting to a loss. The loss may be physical (such as a death), social (such as divorce), or occupational (such as a job). Emotional reactions of grief can include anger, guilt, anxiety , sadness, and despair. Physical reactions of grief can include sleeping problems, changes in appetite, physical problems, or illness.

Group therapy: 1) A type of psychiatric care in which several patients meet with one or more therapists at the same time. The patients form a support group for each other as well as receiving expert care and advice. The group therapy model is particularly appropriate for psychiatric illnesses that are support-intensive, such as anxiety disorders, but is not well suited for treatment of some other psychiatric disorders. 2) A type of psychoanalysis in which patients analyze each other with the assistance of one or more psychotherapists, as in an "encounter group."

Growing pains:Mysterious pains in growing children, usually in the legs. These pains are similar to what the weekend gardener suffers from on Monday-an overuse type of problem. If in playing, children exceed their regular threshold, they will be sore, just like an adult. Growing pains are typically somewhat diffuse (vs. focal) and are not associated with physical changes of the area (such as swelling, redness, etc.).

Heart: The muscle that pumps blood received from veins into arteries throughout the body. It is positioned in the chest behind the sternum (breastbone; in front of the trachea, esophagus, and aorta; and above the diaphragm muscle that separates the chest and abdominal cavities. The normal heart is about the size of a closed fist, and weighs about 10.5 ounces. It is cone-shaped, with the point of the cone pointing down to the left. Two-thirds of the heart lies in the left side of the chest with the balance in the right chest.

Herbal:

- 1. An adjective, referring to herbs, as in an herbal tea.
- 2. A noun, usually reflecting the botanical or medicinal aspects of herbs; also a book which catalogs and illustrates herbs.

The word "herbal" was pronounced with a silent "h" on both sides of the Atlantic until the 19th century but this usage persists only on the American side.

HIV: Acronym for the Human Immunodeficiency Virus , the cause of AIDS (acquired immunodeficiency syndrome). HIV has also been called the human lymphotropic virus type III, the lymphadenopathy-associated virus and the lymphadenopathy virus . No matter what name is applied, it is a retrovirus. (A retrovirus has an RNA genome and a reverse transcriptase enzyme. Using the reverse transcriptase , the virus uses its RNA as a template for making complementary DNA which can integrate into the DNA of the host organism).

Homicide:

- 1. The killing of a person.
- 2. Strictly speaking, the killing of a man. femicide . From the Latin meaning murderer, from homo, man + caedere, to kill.

Hormone: A chemical substance produced in the body that controls and regulates the activity of certain cells or organs.

Human immunodeficiency virus : HIV, the cause of AIDS. HIV has also been called the human lymphotropic virus type III, the lymphadenopathy-associated virus and the lymphadenopathy virus. No matter what name is applied, it is a retrovirus. (A retrovirus has an RNA genome and a reverse transcriptase enzyme. Using the reverse transcriptase, the virus uses its RNA as a template for making complementary DNA which can integrate into the DNA of the host organism). Although the American research Robert Gallo at the National Institutes of Health believed he was the first to find HIV, it is now generally accepted that the French physician Luc Montagnier (1932-) and his team at the Pasteur Institute discovered HIV in 1983- 84.

195

Hyperglycemia: A high blood sugar. An elevated level specifically of the sugar glucose in the blood.

Immunodeficiency: Inability to mount a normal immune response. Immunodeficiency can be due to a genetic disease or acquired as in AIDS due to HIV.

Infection: The growth of a parasitic organism within the body. (A parasitic organism is one that lives on or in another organism and draws its nourishment therefrom.) A person with an infection has another organism (a "germ") growing within him, drawing its nourishment from the person.

Insomnia: The perception or complaint of inadequate or poor-quality sleep because of one or more of the following: difficulty falling asleep; waking up frequently during the night with difficulty returning to sleep; waking up too early in the morning; or unrefreshing sleep. Insomnia is not defined by the number of hours of sleep a person gets or how long it takes to fall asleep. Individuals vary normally in their need for, and their satisfaction with, sleep. Insomnia may cause problems during the day, such as tiredness, a lack of energy, difficulty concentrating, and irritability.

Intervention: The act of intervening, interfering or interceding with the intent of modifying the outcome. In medicine, an intervention is usually undertaken to help treat or cure a condition. For example, early intervention may help children with autism to speak. "Acupuncture as a therapeutic intervention is widely practiced in the United States," according to the National Institutes of Health. From the Latin intervenire, to come between.

Kidney: One of a pair of organs located in the right and left side of the abdomen which clear "poisons" from the blood, regulate acid concentration and maintain water balance in the body by excreting urine. The kidneys are part of the urinary tract. The urine then passes through connecting tubes called "ureters" into the bladder. The bladder stores the urine until it is released during urination.

Laboratory: A place for doing tests and research procedures and preparing chemicals, etc. Although "laboratory" looks very like the Latin "laboratorium" (a place to labor, a work place), the word "laboratory" came from the Latin "elaborare" (to work out, as a problem, and with great pains), as evidenced by the Old English spelling "elaboratory" designating "a place where learned effort was applied to the solution of scientific problems."

Lithium : Lithium carbonate (brand names: Eskalith; Lithobid), a drug used as a mood stabilizer for the treatment of manic/depressive (bipolar) disorder . It prevents or diminishes the intensity of episodes of mania in bipolar patients. Typical symptoms of mania include pressure of speech, motor hyperactivity, reduced need for sleep , flight of ideas, grandiosity, elation, poor judgment, aggressiveness and possibly hostility.

Liver: An organ in the upper abdomen that aids in digestion and removes waste products and worn-out cells from the blood. The liver is the largest solid organ in the body. The liver weighs about three and a half pounds (1.6 kilograms). It measures about 8 inches (20 cm) horizontally (across) and 6.5 inches (17 cm) vertically (down) and is 4.5 inches (12 cm) thick.

Lumbar: Referring to the 5 lumbar vertebrae which are situated below the thoracic vertebrae and above the sacral vertebrae in the spinal column. The 5 lumbar vertebrae are represented by the symbols L1 through L5. There are correspondingly 5 lumbar nerves.

Lupus: A chronic inflammatory condition caused by an autoimmune disease. An autoimmune disease occurs when the body's tissues are attacked by its own immune system. Patients with lupus have unusual antibodies in their blood that are targeted against their own body tissues.

Mania: An abnormally elevated mood state characterized by such symptoms as inappropriate elation, increased irritability, severe insomnia, grandiose notions, increased speed and/or volume of speech, disconnected and racing thoughts, increased sexual desire, markedly increased energy and activity level, poor judgment, and inappropriate social behavior. A mild form in mania that does not require hospitalization is termed hypomania. Mania that also features symptoms of depression ("agitated depression ") is called mixed mania.

Manic: Refers to a mood disorder in which a person seems "high", euphoric, expansive, sometimes agitated, hyperexcitable, with flights of ideas and speech.

Meningitis: Inflammation of the meninges, usually due to a bacterial infection but sometimes from viral, protozoan, or other causes (in some cases the cause cannot be determined).

Migraine: Usually, periodic attacks of headaches on one or both sides of the head. These may be accompanied by nausea, vomiting, increased sensitivity of the eyes to light (photophobia), increased sensitivity to sound (phonophobia), dizziness , blurred vision, cognitive disturbances, and other symptoms. Some migraines do not include headache, and migraines may or may not be preceded by an aura.

Mouth: 1. The upper opening of the digestive tract, beginning with the lips and containing the teeth, gums, and tongue. Foodstuffs are broken down mechanically in the mouth by chewing and saliva is added as a lubricant. Saliva contains amylase, an enzyme that digests starch. 2. Any opening or aperture in the body. The mouth in both senses of the word is also called the os, the Latin word for an opening, or mouth. The o in os is pronounced as in hope. The genitive form of os is oris from which comes the word oral.

MRI: Abbreviation and nickname for magnetic resonance imaging . For more information, see: Magnetic Resonance Imaging ; Paul C. Lauterbur ; Peter Mansfield .

Nausea: Nausea, is the urge to vomit. It can be brought by many causes including, systemic illnesses, such as influenza , medications, pain, and inner ear disease. When nausea and/or vomiting are persistent, or when they are accompanied by other severe symptoms such as abdominal pain , jaundice , fever, or bleeding, a physician should be consulted.

Nerve: A bundle of fibers that uses chemical and electrical signals to transmit sensory and motor information from one body part to another. See: Nervous system .

Neurosyphilis: Neurological complications in the third (tertiary) and final phase of syphilis, which involve the central nervous system and can include psychosis, pain, and loss of physical control over a variety of bodily functions.

Onset: In medicine, the first appearance of the signs or symptoms of an illness as, for example, the onset of rheumatoid arthritis . There is always an onset to a disease but never to the return to good health. The default setting is good health.

Outpatient: A patient who is not an inpatient (not hospitalized) but instead is cared for elsewhere -- as in a doctor's office, clinic, or day surgery center. The term outpatient dates back at least to 1715. Outpatient care today is also called ambulatory care .

Pain: An unpleasant sensation that can range from mild, localized discomfort to agony. Pain has both physical and emotional components. The physical part of pain results from nerve stimulation. Pain may be contained to a discrete area, as in an injury, or it can be more diffuse, as in disorders like fibromyalgia . Pain is mediated by specific nerve fibers that carry the pain impulses to the brain where their conscious appreciation may be modified by many factors.

Panic: A sudden strong feeling of fear that prevents reasonable thought or action.

Panic disorder : A disorder characterized by sudden attacks of fear and panic. The episodes may resemble a heart attack . They may strike at any time and occur without a known reason but more frequently are triggered by specific events or thoughts, such as taking an elevator or driving. The attacks may be so terrifying that some people associate their attacks with the place they occurred and will refuse to go there again.

Pharmacy: A location where prescription drugs are sold. A pharmacy is, by law, constantly supervised by a licensed pharmacist.

Phobia: An unreasonable sort of fear that can cause avoidance and panic. Phobias are a relatively common type of anxiety disorder.

Pregnancy : The state of carrying a developing embryo or fetus within the female body. This condition can be indicated by positive results on an over-the-counter urine test, and confirmed through a blood test, ultrasound, detection of fetal heartbeat, or an X-ray. Pregnancy lasts for about nine months, measured from the date of the woman's last menstrual period (LMP). It is conventionally divided into three trimesters, each roughly three months long.

Pregnant: The state of carrying a developing fetus within the body.

Prescription: A physician's order for the preparation and administration of a drug or device for a patient. A prescription has several parts. They include the superscription or heading with the symbol "R" or "Rx", which stands for the word recipe (meaning, in Latin, to take); the inscription, which contains the names and quantities of the ingredients; the subscription or directions for compounding the drug; and the signature which is often preceded by the sign "s" standing for signa (Latin for mark), giving the directions to be marked on the container.

Psychiatric: Pertaining to or within the purview of psychiatry , the medical specialty concerned with the prevention, diagnosis , and treatment of mental illness.

Psychiatrist: A physician (an M.D.) who specializes in the prevention , diagnosis, and treatment of mental illness . Psychiatrists must receive additional training and serve a supervised residency in their specialty. They may also have additional training in a psychiatric specialty, such as child psychiatry or neuropsychiatry. They can prescribe medication, which psychologists cannot do.

Psychiatry: The medical specialty concerned with the prevention, diagnosis , and treatment of mental illness.

Psychosis: In the general sense, a mental illness that markedly interferes with a person's capacity to meet life's everyday demands. In a specific sense, it refers to a thought disorder in which reality testing is grossly impaired.

Psychotherapy: The treatment of a behavior disorder, mental illness, or any other condition by psychological means. Psychotherapy may utilize insight, persuasion, suggestion, reassurance, and instruction so that patients may see themselves and their problems more realistically and have the desire to cope effectively with them.

Rash : Breaking out (eruption) of the skin. Medically, a rash is referred to as an exanthem.

Relapse: The return of signs and symptoms of a disease after a patient has enjoyed a remission . For example, after treatment a patient with cancer of the colon went into remission with no sign or symptom of the tumor, remained in remission for 4 years, but then suffered a relapse and had to be treated once again for colon cancer.

Rule out: A term much used in medicine, meaning to eliminate or exclude something from consideration. The ACB (albumin cobalt binding) test helps rule out a heart attack in the differential diagnosis of severe chest pain.

Scan: As a noun, the data or image obtained from the examination of organs or regions of the body by gathering information with a sensing device.

Schizoaffective disorder: A mood disorder that is coupled with some symptoms resembling those of schizophrenia , particularly loss of personality (flat affect) and/or social withdrawal.

Schizophrenia : One of several brain diseases whose symptoms that may include loss of personality (flat affect), agitation, catatonia, confusion, psychosis , unusual behavior, and withdrawal. The illness usually begins in early adulthood.

Seizure: Uncontrolled electrical activity in the brain, which may produce a physical convulsion, minor physical signs, thought disturbances, or a combination of symptoms.

Serotonin: A hormone , also called 5-hydroxytryptamine , in the pineal gland , blood platelets, the digestive tract, and the brain. Serotonin acts both as a chemical messenger that transits nerve signals between nerve cells and that causes blood vessels to narrow.

Sexually transmitted disease: Any disease transmitted by sexual contact; caused by microorganisms that survive on the skin or mucus membranes of the genital area; or transmitted via semen, vaginal secretions, or blood during intercourse. Because the genital areas provide a moist, warm environment that is especially conducive to the proliferation of bacteria, viruses, and yeasts, a great many diseases can be transmitted this way. They include AIDS, chlamydia, genital herpes, genital warts , gonorrhea, syphilis, yeast infections, and some forms of hepatitis. Also known as a morbus venereus or venereal disease.

Sleep : The body's rest cycle.

Social phobia: Excessive fear of embarrassment in social situations that is extremely intrusive and can have debilitating effects on personal and professional relationships.

Sodium: The major positive ion (cation) in fluid outside of cells. The chemical notation for sodium is Na+. When combined with chloride, the resulting substance is table salt.

Spinal tap: Also known as a lumbar puncture or "LP", a spinal tap is a procedure whereby spinal fluid is removed from the spinal canal for the purpose of diagnostic testing. It is particularly helpful in the diagnosis of inflammatory diseases of the central nervous system, especially infections, such as meningitis. It can also provide clues to the diagnosis of stroke , spinal cord tumor and cancer in the central nervous system.

Stress: Forces from the outside world impinging on the individual. Stress is a normal part of life that can help us learn and grow. Conversely, stress can cause us significant problems.

Substance:

1. 1. Material with particular features, as a pressor substance .
2. 2. The material that makes up an organ or structure. Also known in medicine as the substantia.
3. 3. A psychoactive drug as, for example, in substance abuse .

Substance abuse: The excessive use of a substance, especially alcohol or a drug. (There is no universally accepted definition of substance abuse.)

Suicidal: Pertaining to suicide . the taking of ones own life. As in a suicidal gesture, suicidal thought, or suicidal act. An "online lifeline for suicidal undergrads" may help prevent college students from committing suicide.

Suicide prevention: Diminishing the risk of suicide . It may not be possible to eliminate entirely the risk of suicide but it is possible to reduce this risk. For example, the suicide rate among US Air Force personnel fell precipitously after the service launched a community-based suicide prevention program. Suicide should not be viewed solely as a medical or mental health problem, since protective factors such as social support and connectedness appear to play significant roles in the prevention of suicide.

Surgeon: A physician who treats disease, injury, or deformity by operative or manual methods. A medical doctor specialized in the removal of organs, masses and tumors and in doing other procedures using a knife (scalpel). The definition of a "surgeon" has begun to blur in recent years as surgeons have begun to minimize the cutting, employ new technologies that are "minimally invasive," use scopes, etc.

Syndrome: A set of signs and symptoms that tend to occur together and which reflect the presence of a particular disease or an increased chance of developing a particular disease.

Syphilis: A sexually transmitted disease caused by Treponema pallidum, a microscopic organism called a spirochete. This worm-like, spiral-shaped organism infects people by burrowing into the moist mucous membranes of the mouth or genitals. From there, the spirochete produces a non-painful ulcer known as a chancre. There are three stages of syphilis:

Systemic: Affecting the entire body. A systemic disease such as diabetes can affect the whole body. Systemic chemotherapy employs drugs that travel through the bloodstream and reach and affect cells all over the body.

Therapy: The treatment of disease .

Thyroid:

1. The thyroid gland . Also, pertaining to the thyroid gland.
2. A preparation of the thyroid gland used to treat hypothyroidism .
3. Shaped like a shield. (The thyroid gland was so-named by Thomas Wharton in 1656 because it was shaped like an ancient Greek shield.)

Tongue: The tongue is a strong muscle anchored to the floor of the mouth. It is covered by the lingual membrane which has special areas to detect tastes.

Trauma: Any injury , whether physically or emotionally inflicted. "Trauma" has both a medical and a psychiatric definition. Medically, "trauma" refers to a serious or critical bodily injury, wound, or shock . This definition is often associated with trauma medicine practiced in emergency rooms and represents a popular view of the term. In psychiatry , "trauma" has assumed a different meaning and refers to an experience that is emotionally painful, distressful, or shocking, which often results in lasting mental and physical effects.

Tremor: Any abnormal repetitive shaking movement of the body. Tremors have many causes and can be inherited, be related to illnesses such as thyroid disease , or caused by fever , hypothermia, drugs or fear.

Trigger: Something that either sets off a disease in people who are genetically predisposed to developing the disease, or that causes a certain symptom to occur in a person who has a disease. For example, sunlight can trigger rashes in people with lupus .

Tumor: An abnormal mass of tissue. Tumors are a classic sign of inflammation, and can be benign or malignant (cancerous). There are dozens of different types of tumors. Their names usually reflect the kind of tissue they arise in, and may also tell you something about their shape or how they grow. For example, a medulloblastoma is a tumor that arises from embryonic cells (a blastoma) in the inner part of the brain (the medulla). Diagnosis depends on the type and location of the tumor. Tumor marker tests and imaging may be used; some tumors can be seen (for example, tumors on the exterior of the skin) or felt (palpated with the hands).

Urine: Liquid waste. The urine is a clear, transparent fluid. It normally has an amber color. The average amount of urine excreted in 24 hours is from 40 to 60 ounces (about 1,200 cubic centimeters). Chemically, the urine is mainly an aqueous (watery) solution of salt (sodium chloride) and substances called urea and uric acid. Normally, it contains about 960 parts of water to 40 parts of solid matter. Abnormally, it may contain sugar (in diabetes), albumen (a protein) (as in some forms of kidney disease), bile pigments (as in jaundice), or abnormal quantities of one or another of its normal components.

Virus: A microorganism smaller than a bacteria, which cannot grow or reproduce apart from a living cell. A virus invades living cells and uses their chemical machinery to keep itself alive and to replicate itself. It may reproduce with fidelity or with errors (mutations)-this ability to mutate is responsible for the ability of some viruses to change slightly in each infected person, making treatment more difficult.

Withdrawal symptoms: Abnormal physical or psychological features that follow the abrupt discontinuation of a drug that has the capability of producing physical dependence. Common withdrawal symptoms include sweating, tremor , vomiting, anxiety , insomnia , and muscle pain .

BIBLIOGRAPHY

Altshuler LL: Bipolar disorder: are repeated episodes associated with neuroanatomic and cognitive changes? Biol Psychiatry 33:563-565,1993

Altshuler LL, Gitlin MJ, Mintz J, et al: Subsyndromal depression is associated with functional impairment in patients with bipolar disorder. J Clin Psychiatry 63:807-811, 2002

Altshuler L, Suppes T, Black D, et al: Impact of antidepressant discontinuation after acute bipolar depression remission on rates of depressive relapse at 1-year follow-up. Am J Psychiatry 160:1252-1262, 2003

Anthony JC, Folstein M, Romanoski AJ: Comparison of lay DIS and a standardized psychiatric diagnosis. Arch Gen Psychiatry 42:667-675,1985

Baer L: Behavior therapy: endogenous serotonin therapy? J Clin Psychiatry 57 (suppl 6):33-35,1996

Calabrese J, Bowden C, Sachs G, et al: A placebo-controlled 18-month trial of lamotrigine and lithium maintenance treatment in recently depressed patients with bipolar I disorder. J Clin Psychiatry 64:1013-1024,2003

Calabrese JR, Keck PE Jr, MacFadden W, et al: A randomized, double-blind, placebo-controlled trial of quetiapine in the treatment of bipolar I or II depression.

Am J Psychiatry 162:1351-1360,2005

Cipriani A, Barbui C, Geddes JR: Suicide, depression, and antidepressants. Br Med J 330:373-374,2005

Colom F, Vieta E, Martinez-Aran A, et al: A randomized trial on the efficacy of group psychoeducation in the prophylaxis of recurrences in bipolar patients whose disease is in remission. Arch Gen Psychiatry 60:402-407,2003

Das AK, Olfson M, Gameroff MJ, et al: Screening for bipolar disorder in a primary care practice. J Am Med Assoc 293:956-963, 2005

Elkin I, Shea MT, Watkins JT, et al: National Institute of Mental Health Treatment of Depression Collaborative Research Program: general effectiveness of treatments. Arch Gen Psychiatry 46:971-982,1989

Fanelli RJ, McNamara JO: Effects of age on kindling and kindled seizure-induced increase of benzodiazepine receptor binding. Brain Res 362:17-22,1986

Frank E, Kupfer DJ, Perel JM, et al: Three-year outcomes for maintenance therapies in recurrent depression. Arch Gen Psychiatry 47:1093-1099,1990

Ghaemi SN, Rosenquist KJ: Is insight in mania state-dependent? A meta-analysis.
J Nery Ment Dis 192:771-775, 2004

Ghaemi SN, Boiman EE, Goodwin FK: Diagnosing bipolar disorder and the effect of antidepressants: a naturalistic study. J Clin Psychiatry 61:804-808, 2000

Ghaemi SN, Lenox MS, Baldessarini RJ: Effectiveness and safety of long-term antidepressant treatment in bipolar disorder. J Clin Psychiatry 62:565-569, 2001

Ghaemi SN, Hsu DJ, Soldani F, et al: Antidepressants in bipolar disorder: the case for caution. Bipolar Disord 5:421-433,2003

Ghaemi SN, El-Mallakh RS, Baldassano CF, et al: A randomized clinical trial of efficacy and safety of long-term antidepressant use in bipolar disorder (abstract). Bipolar Disord 7 (suppl 2): 59,2005

Gijsman HJ, Geddes JR, Rendell JM, et al: Antidepressants for bipolar depression: a systematic review of randomized, controlled trials. Am J Psychiatry 161:1537-1547, 2004

Goldapple K, Segal Z, Garson C, et al: Modulation of cortical-limbic pathways in major depression: treatment-specific effects of cognitive behavior therapy. Arch Gen Psychiatry 61:34-41,2004

Goodwin FK, Jamison KR: Manic Depressive Illness. New York, Oxford University Press, 1990

Gynther BD, Calford MB, Sah P: Neuroplasticity and psychiatry. Aust N Z J Psychiatry 32:119-128,1998

Hirschfeld RM, Williams JB, Spitzer RL, et al: Development and validation of a screening instrument for bipolar spectrum disorder: the Mood Disorder Questionnaire. Am J Psychiatry 157:1873-1875, 2000

Hirschfeld, RM, Calabrese JR, Weissman MM, et al: Screening for bipolar disorder in the community. J Clin Psychiatry 64:53-59, 2003

Kandel ER: Biology and the future of psychoanalysis: a new intellectual framework
for psychiatry revisited. Am J Psychiatry 156:505-524,1999

Kendler KS, Neale MC, Kessler RC, et al: Childhood parental loss and adult psychopathology in women. A twin study perspective. Arch Gen Psychiatry 49:109-116,1992

Kendler KS, McGuire M, Gruenberg AM: The Roscommon family study, I: methods, diagnosis of probands, and risk of schizophrenia in relatives. Arch Gen Psychiatry 50:527-540,1993a

Kendler KS, Walters EE, Neale MC: The structure of the genetic and environmental risk factors for six major psychiatric disorders in women. Arch Gen Psychiatry 52:374-383,1993b

Kendler KS, Gallagher TJ, Abelson JM, et al: Lifetime prevalence, demographic risk factors, and diagnostic validity of nonaffective psychosis as assessed in a US community sample: the national comorbidity survey. Arch Gen Psychiatry 53:1022-1031,1996

Kessler RC, McGonagle KA, Zhao S: Lifetime and 12-month prevalence of DSM-III-R psychiatric disorders in the United States. Arch Gen Psychiatry 51:8-19,1994

Lampe 1K, Hulshoff Pol HE, Janssen J, et al: Association of depression duration with reduction of global cerebral gray matter volume in female patients with recurrent major depressive disorder. Am J Psychiatry 160:2052-2054, 2003

Manji HK: G proteins: implications for psychiatry. Am J Psychiatry 149:746-760, 1992

Martinez-Aran A, Vieta E, Colom F, et al: Cognitive impairment in euthymic bipolar patients: implications for clinical and functional outcome. Bipolar Disord 6:224-232,2004

Mayberg HS: Positron emission tomography imaging in depression: a neural systems perspective. Neuroimaging Clin N Am 13:805-815, 2003

Mayberg HS, Lozano AM, Voon V, et al: Deep brain stimulation for treatmentresistant depression. Neuron 45:651-660, 2005

Miklowitz D, Craighead W: Bipolar affective disorder: does psychosocial treatment add to the efficacy of drug therapy? Economics of Neuroscience 3:58-64, 2001

Nemeroff CB, Evans DL, Gyulai L, et al: Double-blind, placebo-controlled comparison of imipramine and paroxetine in the treatment of bipolar depression. Am J Psychiatry 158:906-912,2001

Papolos DF, Veit S, Faedda GL, et al: Ultra-ultra rapid cycling bipolar disorder is associated with the low activity catecholamine-O-methyltransferase allele. Mol Psychiatry 3:346-349,1998

Post RM: The transduction of psychosocial stress into the neurobiology of recurrent affective illness. Am J Psychiatry 149:999-1010,1992

Post R, Altshuler L, Leverich G, et al: Randomized comparison of bupropion, sertraline, and venlafaxine as adjunctive treatment in acute bipolar depression, in Program and Abstracts, American Psychiatric Association 157th Annual Meeting, New York, May 1-6,2004. Washington, DC, American

Psychiatric Association, 2004, pp 259-265

Rousseva A, Henry C, van den Bulke D, et al: Antidepressant-induced mania, rapid cycling and the serotonin transporter gene polymorphism. Pharmacogenomics J 3:101-104,2003

Thase ME: The clinical, psychosocial, and pharmacoeconomic ramifications of remission. Am J Manag Care 7:S377-S385, 2001

Thase ME, Sloan DM, Kornstein SG: Remission as the critical outcome of depression treatment. Psychopharmacol Bull 36:12-25,2002

Tohen M, Hennen J, Zarate CJ, et al: The McLean first episode project: two-year syndromal and functional recovery in 219 cases of major affective disorders with psychotic features. Am J Psychiatry 157:220-228,2000

Tohen M, Vieta E, Calabrese J, et al: Efficacy of olanzapine and olanzapinefluoxetine combination in the treatment of bipolar I depression. Arch Gen Psychiatry 60:1079-1088,2003

van Gorp WG, Altshuler L, Theberge DC, et al: Cognitive impairment in euthymic bipolar patients with and without prior alcohol dependence. A preliminary study. Arch Gen Psychiatry 55:41-46,1998

Wehr TA, Goodwin FK: Biological rhythms in manic-depressive illness, in Circadian Rhythms in Psychiatry. Edited by Wehr TA, Goodwin FK. Pacific Grove, CA, Boxwood Press, 1983, pp 129-184